DRS. JORDAN'S ™ WHATS, WHYS and HOWS ™

RATIONALES of ™ CARDIOLOGY

BOOK ONE: CARDIOVASCULAR SYSTEM

DRS. JORDAN'S ™
WHATS, WHYS and HOWS ™

RATIONALES of ™
CARDIOLOGY

BOOK ONE:
CARDIOVASCULAR SYSTEM

James L. Jordan, PhD, PhD
and
Deovina N. Jordan, PhD, MD

Copyright Page

Title: DRS. JORDAN'S ™ WHATS, WHYS and HOWS ™
RATIONALES OF ™ CARDIOLOGY
BOOK ONE: CARDIOVASCULAR SYSTEM

Paperback ISBN-13: 978-1-64752-026-7
EBook ISBN-13: 978-1-64752-027-4

If you have any questions about the content of this book, please contact Deja Jord, Inc.
23811 Washington Avenue, C110, #249
Murrieta, California 92562

Dedication

We dedicate this book to:

All Who Thirst For Knowledge

James L. Jordan, PhD, PhD

and

Deovina N. Jordan, PhD, MD

Prologue

This book is the product of three decades of research into what, why and how different things occur in healthcare and why healthcare practitioners do what they do. Needless to say, the information is extensive and widely dispersed, and, as a consequence, not easy to obtain. While there is an abundance of facts, namely the "whats" in medicine, nursing, and other healthcare professions, there is much less information available about the rationales or the "whys" and "hows" of things in the healthcare professions. But, knowing why and how something happens helps one to know what to do and what needs to be learned/ researched/ developed. And, just as important, that means this kind of work will always be a work in progress. As healthcare knowledge improves, so does our understanding. And, as our healthcare understanding advances, so do our questions. Finally, as our questions change, so does our healthcare knowledge base change as we answer, or seek to answer, those questions.

The published literature on healthcare abounds in presentations of information focused on a plethora of facts. The authors wholeheartedly believe that these sources of information are invaluable in healthcare practice and understanding. Also, other publications often address current healthcare theories and hypotheses. These will help healthcare practitioners understand what the current thought and research trends are. However, healthcare theories and hypotheses are not addressed in this book as they often change with the times and, more importantly, they are not the foci of this book.

Because this book addresses both "whats" and "whys", and "whats" and "hows," it has been arranged not only by topic but also according to statements. The "what" statements are mentioned first. Then the "why" or "how" statements follow. The authors acknowledge a certain lack of continuity that would be present if only facts or "whats" are presented. To the authors' knowledge, this is the first time such an attempt to systematically address "whats" and their "whys" or "hows" have been made. Considering the time utilized and the efforts expended to obtain the information included in this book, along with the vast sea of information which needed to be reviewed in order to glean these pearls of understanding, this is quite understandable. Few people would have gone on a thirty year journey, surveying thousands of documents, without knowing where it would lead them.

This book is about the "Whats," "Whys" and "Hows" or Rationales of Cardiology. Book One focuses on the Cardiovascular System and is specifically about Blood Flow; Blood Pressure, Hypertension (Different Types) and Hypotension; Blood Supply, Blood Volume and Circulation; Peripheral Circulation, Deep Vein/Venous Thrombosis, Peripheral Arterial Disease, and Peripheral Vascular Disease; Pulmonary Circulation and Pulmonary Embolism;

Thromboembolism, Thrombophlebitis and Thrombosis; and Disseminated Intravascular Coagulation. Pulmonary circulation was included as part of the cardiovascular system. Some topics may be repeated in different sections due to the overlap of disorders when discussing the cardiovascular system. Topics within the chapters are arranged alphabetically. The information presented in this book reflects the latest in literature as of publication date.

Finally, this is not a book written to provide medical, nursing, or any other healthcare advice. This book is in no way a substitute for well-trained healthcare professionals practicing in their fields of expertise.

Table of Contents

Chapter 1: Blood Flow

Blood Flow -- Brain (Cerebral)

Syncope is the transient loss of consciousness and postural tone.

> Reason: Loss of consciousness and postural tone during syncope occurs due to inadequate cerebral blood flow.

Confusion, syncope, slowed speech and thinking, and memory loss may occur with hypothyroidism.

> Reason: Decreased cerebral blood flow in hypothyroidism leads to cerebral hypoxia - causing the above signs and symptoms.

Death may occur from herniation of intracranial contents.

> Reason: Death results from cessation of cerebral blood flow and respirations.

Regional hypoxia leading to cell death occurs with prolonged seizures.

> Reason: Prolonged seizures cause uncoupling of cerebral blood flow and metabolic demand.

Brain swelling reduces cerebral blood flow.

> Reason: The brain is enclosed in a rigid structure (the skull).

Fluctuating and often bizarre neurological abnormalities occur with thrombolytic thrombocytopenic purpura.

> Reason: Due to interruption of blood flow to the brain.

Cerebral arteries dilate with malignant hypertension (HTN).

> Reason: Markedly elevated blood pressure causes decompensation of the normal autoregulation of cerebral blood flow.

Brain stem herniation may result in brain anoxia and death.

> Reason: Cessation of blood flow results from increased pressure on the brain stem.

Cardiac stimulants may cause headaches.

> Reason: Due to dilation of cerebral blood vessels.

Restlessness, agitation, or confusion occurs in early cardiogenic shock.

Reason: Decreased cardiac output results in decreased cerebral blood flow.

Sudden decrease in blood pressure in a hypertensive individual can be detrimental.

Reason: Too sudden and/or too great of a reduction in blood pressure can reduce the body's ability to autoregulate cerebral blood flow.

Blood Flow -- Capillary

Multiple myeloma, Waldenstrom's macroglobinemia and cryoglobulinemia can lead to retinal hemorrhages.

Reasons: Proteins cause markedly increased serum viscosity and impaired blood flow through the capillaries.

Diabetics have decreased microvascular flow.

Reason: Due to abnormalities in diabetic red blood cells.

Blood Flow -- Coronary

Coronary blood flow diminishes with aortic stenosis.

Reason: Because of high intracavity pressures.

With coronary artery disease, coronary blood flow becomes inadequate to meet metabolic needs.

Reason: Progressive compromise in coronary blood flow (usually from development of atherosclerotic plaques).

Blood Flow -- Decreased

The skin is cool with hypothyroidism.

Reason: From decreased blood flow.

Food intolerance is an age-related change.

Reasons: Because of (1) gastric mucosa atrophy and (2) blood flow decrease.

Decreased blood flow in the small arteries and limited venous return occurs with compartment syndrome.

Reason: The fascia limits outward swelling; as such, the inflammation is directed inward.

Microaneurysms and irregular flow patterns (diminishing blood flow) occur in individuals with diabetes.

Reason: Thickening of the basement membranes.

Portal HTN is a factor that leads the development of ascites.

Reason: Increased resistance of blood flow through the liver.

Prolonged bed rest is contraindicated postoperatively in individuals who have undergone ligation and stripping.

Reasons: Because of (1) decreased blood flow to the heart and (2) venous stasis.

Hypovolemia is a factor that may precipitate hepatic encephalopathy.

Reasons: (1) Increased blood ammonia causing hepatic hypoxia and (2) impaired cerebral, hepatic and renal functions from decreased blood flow.

Blood Flow -- Doppler Assessment

Sound cannot be detected by Doppler ultrasound in totally occluded blood vessels.

Reason: Doppler ultrasound amplifies the sound generated by vascular blood flow.

Blood Flow -- Fetal

A fetus has low pulmonary blood flow.

Reason: Because of high pulmonary vascular resistance.

Blood Flow -- Increased

Increased blood flow in the skin, particularly in the hands and feet, occurs during pregnancy.

Reasons: Peripheral vasodilation and increased numbers of capillaries.

Increased blood flow and capillary permeability occur with rheumatoid arthritis.

Reason: Because of inflammatory response.

Blood Flow -- Impaired

Impaired blood flow occurs with polycythemia.

Reasons: Due to hypervolemia and hyperviscosity.

Blood Flow -- Local

Heat applied to the skin increases local blood flow.

Reason: Because of vasodilation.

Blood Flow -- Muscles

Major changes in muscular blood flow and cardiac output occur during exercise.

Reasons: Due to reflex compensatory activity from central commands and muscle vasodilation.

A reduced ability to perform aerobic exercise is a hallmark of heart failure.

Reason: Inadequate blood flow to active skeletal muscles secondary to impaired cardiac output.

Blood Flow -- Obstruction

Sudden death may occur with atrial myxoma.

Reasons: From (1) coronary embolization, (2) systemic embolization, (3) obstruction of blood flow from the mitral valve, and/or (4) obstruction of blood flow from the tricuspid valve.

Blood Flow -- Pooling

Prolonged standing can lead to diminished intracardiac volume.

Reason: From pooling of blood in the lower extremities.

An increase in pooling of blood in the right ventricle occurs with status asthmaticus.

Reason: A significant increase in negative intrapleural pressure results from increased muscle force.

Blood Flow -- Pregnancy

Increased blood flow in the skin, particularly in the hands and feet, occurs during pregnancy.

Reasons: Because of peripheral vasodilation and increased numbers of capillaries.

Blood Flow -- Pulmonary

In mitral stenosis, pulmonary blood flow eventually decreases, which then decreases systemic blood flow.

Reason: Due to failure of the right ventricle.

Pulmonary circulation affects the blood composition supplying all organs.

Reason: All cardiac output goes through the lungs before entering the systemic circulation.

Pulmonary blood flow is not uniformly distributed throughout a lung.

Reason: Due to gravity dependence from regional differences in pulmonary vascular pressure and resistance.

The right side of the heart may become strained in severe cases of beryliosis.

Reason: Lung damage (including scarring) causes increased pressure in the pulmonary artery.

Symptoms of large-sized ventricular septal defects (VSD) may be delayed.

Reason: From delayed decrease in pulmonary vascular pressures.

Symptoms of medium-sized VSD occur earlier in premature infants than in full-term infants.

Reason: Pulmonary resistance decreases earlier in preterm infants than in full-term infants.

Forced lung inflation causes increased right ventricular afterload.

Reason: Due to the increased intrathoracic pressure compressing the pulmonary microcirculation.

No blood flows through the fetal pulmonary artery.

Reason: The collapsed fetal lung, which is not used for breathing during pregnancy, has virtually infinite vascular resistance.

In a fetus, 90% of the pulmonary arterial blood bypasses the lung.

Reason: Due to shunting that occurs through the ductus arteriosus (because of the high vascular resistance in the lungs).

With the first few breaths, the neonates' deoxygenated blood returns to the right ventricle and then to the lungs to become oxygenated.

Reasons: Because of (1) falling pulmonary vascular resistance, (2) closure of the foramen ovale and (3) constriction of the ductus arteriosus.

Blood Flow -- Redistribution

Portal HTN can lead to increased production of aldosterone.

Reasons: Due to reduced renal perfusion and blood flow redistribution.

Blood Flow -- Renal

Decreased glomerular filtration rate (GFR) occurs with hypothyroidism.

Reason: Because of decreased renal blood flow.

Loop diuretics increase renal blood flow.

Reason: Loop diuretics exert a vasodilatory effect on the renal vasculature.

Distal pressures with aortic stenosis are not as low as one would expect from hemodynamics alone.

Reasons: Reduced systemic blood flow (renal blood flow in particular) causes increased renin release and activation of the renin-angiotensin-aldosterone system; elevated blood volume and arterial pressure result.

Glomerular blood flow decreases with acute renal failure.

Reasons: Because of (1) arteriolar vasoconstriction, (2) capillary obstruction by thrombi and (3) endothelial cell edema.

Renal failure (anuria or oliguria) may occur with acute gastrointestinal hemorrhage.

Reasons: From decreased blood flow to the kidneys and acute tubular necrosis.

Portal HTN can lead to redistribution of blood flow (with reduced renal perfusion).

Reason: Because of the persistence of amine neurotransmitters.

Hyperaldosteronism is a factor that leads to the development of ascites.

Reasons: From (1) increased aldosterone secretion stimulated by decreased renal blood flow and (2) increased aldosterone due to impaired liver metabolism

Clonidine may be administered to treat HTN complicated by renal disease.

Reason: Clonidine does not decrease renal blood flow or glomerular filtration.

Renal artery stenosis, as indicated by a renal artery bruit, may lead to either acute or chronic renal dysfunction.

Reason: Due to compromised blood flow to the kidneys.

Decreased renal blood flow occurs with diabetic ketoacidosis (DKA).

Reason: From hypotension.

Blood Flow -- Resistance to

Increased resistance to blood flow occurs with cirrhosis of the liver.

Reason: Enlarged liver cells compress the liver lobule.

Blood Flow -- Stasis

Circulatory stasis occurs with polycythemia.

Reasons: Due to hypervolemia and hyperviscosity of the blood.

Chapter 2: Blood Pressure, Hypertension (Different Types) and Hypotension

Blood Pressure (BP) -- Assessment of

Do not take blood pressure (BP) readings on the arm nearest to a radical mastectomy site.

Reason: Permanent lymphedema may result.

A BP cuff that is too large in relation to a person's arm produces an invalid BP reading.

Reason: The reading is falsely low.

A BP cuff that is too small in relation to a person's arm produces an invalid BP reading.

Reason: The reading is falsely high.

Blood pressure measurements do not assess controllability.

Reason: Blood pressure measurements are made at rest and, therefore, only assess baseline characteristic values.

Blood Pressure (BP) -- Baroreceptors

In spite of being exposed to higher-than-normal BPs, the aortic arch and carotid baroreceptors have a blunted response.

Reasons: (1) Structural changes in the walls of the baroreceptors and (2) desensitization to chronic elevated pressure; thus, setting their norm to a higher pressure.

Blood Pressure (BP) -- Compensatory Mechanisms

Vasoconstriction occurs with diabetic ketoacidosis (DKA).

Reason: It is a compensatory mechanism from fluid volume deficit to preserve BP.

Heart rate increases with septic shock.

Reasons: To compensate for hypotension and reaction to increased metabolism and stimulation of sympathetic nervous system (SNS) and adrenal glands.

Blood Pressure (BP) -- Decreased

At higher doses, nicotine causes a drop in BP.

Reason: From ganglionic blockade.

Blood pressure drops during septic shock.

Reason: Due to reduction of preload and afterload.

Blood Pressure (BP) -- Differences – Upper vs. Lower Extremities

With coarctation of the aorta, bounding pulses and increased BP occur in the upper extremities while decreased (or absent) pulses and decreased BP occur in the lower extremities.

Reason: These result from the narrowing of the aortic arch.

Blood Pressure (BP) -- Distal

With aortic stenosis, distal pressures are not as low as one would expect from hemodynamics alone.

Reasons: Reduced systemic blood flow (renal blood flow in particular) causes increased renin release and activation of the renin-angiotensin-aldosterone system; elevated blood volume and arterial pressure result.

Blood Pressure (BP) -- Hypertension (HTN) – Catecholamine Crisis

Cocaine can cause HTN.

Reason: Due to catecholamine crisis.

Amphetamines can cause HTN.

Reason: Also due to catecholamine crisis.

Monoamine oxidase (MAO) inhibitors and indirect-acting catechols (e.g., wine, cheese, ephedrine) can cause HTN.

Reason: Also due to catecholamine crisis.

Tricyclic antidepressants and direct-acting catechols (e.g., epinephrine, pseudoephedrine, norepinephrine) can cause HTN.

Reason: Also due to catecholamine crisis.

Pheochromocytoma can produce a hypertensive crisis (catecholamine crisis).

Reason: Epinephrine, or norepinephrine, is overproduced.

Blood Pressure (BP) -- Hypertension (HTN) – Comorbidities and Complications

Medullary HTN can occur in osteoarthritis (OA).

Reason: The thickened subchondral trabeculae lead to distortion of blood flow.

Atrial fibrillation produces comorbidities.

Reason: Atrial fibrillation may lead to HTN, pulmonary congestion, or angina pectoris.

Hypertension (HTN) often occurs in patients with angina pectoris.

Reason: A linear relationship exists between left ventricular systolic pressure and myocardial demand; as peripheral vascular resistance increases so does left ventricular systolic pressure.

Hypertension (HTN) occurs with nephritic syndrome.

Reason: Because of salt and water retention.

Individuals with coarctation of the aorta are at increased risk for cerebral aneurysms and hemorrhage.

Reason: Severe HTN.

Hypertension (HTN) may cause heart failure (HF).

Reason: Due to pressure overload.

Individuals with polycystic kidney disease often have high BP.

Reason: Thought to result from renal ischemia from the enlarging cysts.

Note the presence of pedal edema in a hypertensive patient.

Reason: It is indicative of HF or nephrosis.

Note the presence of truncal obesity in a hypertensive patient.

Reason: It is indicative of Cushing's syndrome.

Assess a hypertensive patient for bruits over the renal arteries.

Reason: Their presence is an indication of renal artery stenosis.

Assess the skin of a hypertensive patient for striae.

Reason: Striae are an indication of Cushing's syndrome.

Assess the skin of a hypertensive patient for uremic appearance.

Reason: It is an indication of chronic renal failure (RF).

Renal failure (RF) occurs with thrombotic thrombocytopenic purpura.

Reasons: Due to (1) renal cortical infarction and (2) HTN.

A renin-dependent form of HTN can occur with glomerulonephritis.

Reason: Renal disease may increase the release of renin.

Blurred vision can result from HTN.

Reason: Because of arteriolar changes in the eye.

Hypertension (HTN) must be controlled for individuals with abdominal aortic aneurysms.

Reason: Inherent risks that the weakened vessels will rupture.

About a third of hypertensive persons do not know they have HTN.

Reason: Hypertension (HTN) is usually asymptomatic until organ/ tissue damage has occurred.

Hyperthyroidism can lead to HTN.

Reasons: From (1) induction of systemic vasoconstriction, (2) increased blood volume and (3) increased cardiac activity.

Hypertension (HTN) and volume expansion occur in Cushing's syndrome.

Reason: Because of excessive glucocorticoids.

Sodium and water retention occur in most hypertensive patients.

Reason: Due to alteration in renal function.

Blood volume, cardiac output, and arterial pressure increase in hypertensive patients.

Reason: Alteration in renal function leads to retention of sodium and water.

Among persons with variceal hemorrhage, higher rates of bleeding are reported in those with left-sided portal HTN.

Reason: From thrombosis of the splenic vein.

Hypertension (HTN) is a cause of ischemic heart disease.

Reasons: Due to (1) increased oxygen demand and (2) increased cardiac work.

Heart failure (HF) may occur with RF.

Reasons: From increased fluid volume and chronic HTN.

Individuals with coarctation of the aorta are at increased risk for premature coronary arteriosclerosis.

Reason: Because of severe HTN.

Individuals with coarctation of the aorta are at increased risk for infective endocarditis.

Reason: Due to severe HTN.

Systemic HTN occurs with sleep apnea syndrome.

Reason: This is a consequence of repetitive oxygen desaturation.

Hypertension (HTN) should be treated aggressively in persons with chronic RF.

Reason: Hypertension (HTN) accelerates the rate of renal function decline.

The heart enlarges in individuals with severe HTN.

Reason: The heart enlarges to compensate for increased resistance.

Individuals with coarctation of the aorta are at increased risk for left ventricular failure.

Reason: Because of severe HTN.

Blood Pressure (BP) -- Hypertension (HTN) – Contraindications

Avoid general anesthesia in persons with uncontrolled HTN.

Reason: To minimize risk of catastrophic cerebral events.

Blood Pressure (BP) -- Hypertension (HTN) – Essential, Primary

Symptoms (such as chest discomfort, dizziness, fatigue, headache, palpitations) and their level of intensity are inconsistent with regards to primary (essential) HTN.

Reason: The symptoms above do not correlate well with BP levels. To illustrate, most individuals with primary (essential) HTN are usually asymptomatic.

Blood Pressure (BP) -- Hypertension (HTN) – Faulty or Inappropriate Apparatus

Aneroid sphygmomanometers require regular calibration.

Reason: Since they may lose accuracy with time.

Dirt in the escape valves of aneroid sphygmomanometers can contribute to inaccurate BP readings.

Reason: By causing irregular deflation.

An aneroid sphygmomanometer with a mercury column must read zero before inflation.

Reason: If the mercury column does not read zero before inflation, the reading will be inaccurate as the mercury column at zero reading is the baseline.

An aneroid sphygmomanometer with a mercury column must be vertical.

Reason: A nonvertical mercury column will overestimate the BP.

When using an aneroid sphygmomanometer with a mercury column, keep the eye at the level with the upper level meniscus.

Reason: To prevent erroneous readings due to parallax.

If the rubber bladder (in the sphygmomanometer cuff) is too short, the BP will be overestimated.

Reason: Due to the BP not being fully transmitted to the artery.

Rapid reinflation of the cuff will lead to overestimating the systolic BP level.

Reason: This will increase the level at which the Korotkoff sounds will appear.

Failure to deflate the cuff properly before repeating BP measurements will lead to overestimating the systolic BP level.

Reason: This will also increase the level at which the Korotkoff sounds will appear.

The arm used for BP reading should not be in a dependent position.

Reason: This will cause overestimation of diastolic and systolic pressures. Note: The arm should be supported at the mid-sternal level.

Anxiety can cause an elevation of BP.

Reason: Due to the activation of the autonomic nervous system.

Cold temperature can cause an elevation of BP.

Reason: Also due to the activation of the autonomic nervous system.

Physical pain can cause an elevation of BP.

Reason: Due to the activation of the autonomic nervous system.

Recent cigarette smoking can cause an elevation of BP.

Reason: Also due to the activation of the autonomic nervous system.

Recent physical activity can cause an elevation of BP.

Reason: Due to the activation of the autonomic nervous system.

Blood Pressure (BP) -- Hypertension (HTN) – Intracranial

In individuals with intracranial HTN, avoid chest physiotherapy during periods of poor cerebral compliance.

Reason: To prevent increased intrathoracic pressure.

Visual changes may occur with brain tumors.

Reason: They are caused by papilledema from chronic intracranial HTN.

Anticonvulsant agents are administered prophylactically to persons with increased intracranial pressure.

Reason: Seizures cause blood pressure to increase leading to intracranial HTN.

In individuals with intracranial HTN, maintain body alignment (including hip flexion, neck flexion).

Reason: To prevent cerebral venous drainage obstruction.

Sustained elevated intracranial pressure can be fatal.

Reason: Because of brain stem depression or herniation.

Blood Pressure (BP) -- Hypertension (HTN) – Malignant

Cerebral arteries dilate with malignant HTN.

Reason: From decompensation of the normal autoregulation of cerebral blood flow because of markedly elevated BP.

Blood Pressure (BP) -- Hypertension (HTN) – Physiology

Hypertension (HTN) has been called the "silent killer."

> Reason: Most individuals with arterial HTN are asymptomatic. Yet, arterial HTN can result in adverse, serious cardiovascular problems such as ischemic heart disease, heart failure (HF), myocardial infarction (MI), and stroke.

The absolute level of BP is not the major threat in HTN.

> Reason: The rise in rates of BP is the real hazard. This is borne out of the fact that individuals with chronic HTN are capable of tolerating much higher BPs than persons who are normally normotensive.

Intimal disruption (most often at the edges of plaques) occurs with chronic HTN.

> Reasons: The intimal disruption is a consequence of changes in arterial wall composition (intimal thickening, calcification, fibrosis, extracellular fatty acid deposition) along with changes in the extracellular matrix (accelerated degradation, apoptosis, elastolysis with hyalinization of collagen).

Necrosis of smooth muscle cells in arteries occurs with chronic HTN.

Reasons: This is due to increased intimal thickening (reducing nutrient and oxygen supply to arterial vessel walls), adventitial fibrosis (obstructing vessels which supply nourishment to the arterial wall) and small intramural vasa vasorum.

Fibrosis of elastic structures in arterial walls occurs with chronic HTN.

Reasons: Also, from increased intimal thickening (reducing nutrient and oxygen supply to arterial vessel walls), adventitial fibrosis (obstructing vessels which supply nourishment to the arterial wall) and small intramural vasa vasorum.

Arterial wall stiffness increases with chronic HTN.

Reasons: Due to the necrosis of smooth muscle cells and increased intimal thickening.

Vulnerability to pulsatile forces increases with chronic HTN.

Reasons: From the necrosis of smooth muscle cells and increased intimal thickening.

Individuals with coarctation of the aorta are at increased risk for rupture of the aorta.

Reason: Because of severe HTN.

With stress, cardiac output and blood pressure increase.

Reason: Cortisol levels increase.

Renal retention of sodium and water are necessary to sustain a hypertensive state.

Reason: To increase blood volume.

Blood pressures (BPs) should be closely monitored in renal transplant patients.

Reason: Up to 80% of patients develop HTN.

Increased arteriolar resistance and reduced venous system capacitance occur with HTN.

Reason: Due to increased peripheral vascular smooth muscle tone.

Hypertension (HTN) can result from pain.

Reason: Because of increased catecholamine secretion.

Blood Pressure (BP) -- Hypertension (HTN) – Portal

Portal HTN can cause congestive splenomegaly.

Reason: The splenic vein drains into the portal vein.

Portal HTN can lead to increased production of aldosterone.

Reason: Redistribution of blood flow (in reduced renal perfusion).

Portal HTN can lead to persistence of amine neurotransmitters.

Reason: Collateral venous vessels develop.

Portal HTN can lead to transudation of plasma into the abdominal cavity.

Reason: Because of vasocongestion within the intestinal vasculature.

Portal HTN can lead to increased sodium and water retention.

Reason: Due to increased aldosterone production.

Portal HTN can lead to dilation of lymph channels draining the liver.

Reason: From increased liver lymph (high protein) production.

Portal HTN can lead to increased leakage of plasma from the liver tissues into the abdominal cavity.

Reason: Plasma leaks out of the vasculature from the liver tissues eventually leaking and affecting the abdominal cavity.

Increase in portal venous pressure (portal HTN) occurs with esophagogastric varices.

Reason: Inadequate liver sinusoid function causes increased portal blood flow and elevated pressures within the liver.

Portal HTN is a factor that leads to the development of ascites.

Reason: Due to increased resistance of blood flow through the liver.

Nonselective beta-blockers reduce portal pressure.

Reasons: By decreasing cardiac output and splanchnic vasoconstriction.

Blood Pressure (BP) -- Hypertension (HTN) – Pregnancy

Hypertension (HTN) decreases uteroplacental blood flow.

Reason: Due to maternal vasoconstriction.

Elevated arterial pressure should be reduced slowly when treating preeclampsia.

Reasons: To avoid hypotension and decreased blood flow to the fetus.

Cerebral ischemia may occur with preeclampsia/ eclampsia.

Reason: Because of HTN.

Complete blood count is a laboratory test used in the assessment of pregnant hypertensive patients.

Reason: Increasing hematocrit may indicate worsening vasoconstriction and decreased intravascular volume.

Platelet count is a laboratory test used in the assessment of pregnant hypertensive patients.

Reason: Because of the association of thrombocytopenia and coagulopathy with worsening pregnancy induced HTN (PIH).

Assess for right upper quadrant pain in a pregnant patient with HTN.

Reason: It is indicative of hepatic congestion.

Preeclampsia differs from less severe forms of PIH

Reasons: It is worse because of (1) renal damage resulting in loss of albumin in the urine and (2) significant systemic edema.

Liver function studies are used in the assessment of pregnant patients with HTN.

Reason: Hepatocellular dysfunction is associated with worsening PIH.

Diuretics should not be administered to a patient with PIH.

Reasons: Hypovolemia and fetal distress may result.

Salt should not be restricted in a patient with PIH.

Reasons: Hypovolemia and fetal distress may also result.

Blood Pressure (BP) -- Hypertension (HTN), Pulmonary – Pathophysiology

The term "primary pulmonary HTN (PPH)" is no longer used.

Reason: The new term is "idiopathic pulmonary arterial HTN (IPAH)."

In healthy individuals (e.g., those without pulmonary HTN), increases in pulmonary blood flow, induced by exercise, result in minor increases in pulmonary arterial pressure.

Reason: Due to a decrease in pulmonary vascular resistance.

In healthy individuals (e.g., those without pulmonary HTN), pulmonary vascular resistance decreases with exercise-related increases in pulmonary blood flow.

Reason: From the utilization of previously unperfused as well as already perfused pulmonary vessels.

Pulmonary HTN can result in decreased cardiac index.

Reason: Because of increased afterload.

Blood Pressure (BP) -- Hypertension (HTN), Pulmonary – Pathophysiology – Early Stages

In the early stages of pulmonary HTN, pulmonary arterial pressure is normal at rest, but elevated with exercise.

Reasons: Due to the (1) loss of the pulmonary vascular bed to dilate and (2) the inability to utilize unused vasculature; however, the right ventricle (RV) hypertrophies.

In the early stages of pulmonary HTN, the right ventricle hypertrophies.

Reason: In response to increased afterload.

Blood Pressure (BP) -- Hypertension (HTN), Pulmonary – Pathophysiology – Progression of

As pulmonary HTN progresses, the right heart diastolic pressure and the right atrial pressure both increase.

> Reason: As right ventricular failure develops.

Left ventricular end-diastolic and pulmonary capillary wedge pressures increase as pulmonary HTN and right ventricular failure progress.

> Reason: Due to impairment of left ventricular compliance by progressive right ventricular dilation.

Mean pulmonary arterial pressure decreases as right ventricular failure ensues.

> Reason: Impairment of forward flow.

Blood Pressure (BP) -- Hypertension (HTN), Pulmonary – Pathophysiology – Chronic

Right ventricular wall thickness increases (i.e., RV hypertrophy) in chronic pulmonary HTN.

> Reason: To normalize myocardial oxygen consumption and wall stress.

Blood Pressure (BP) -- Hypertension (HTN), Pulmonary – Causes

Anemia can cause pulmonary HTN.

Reason: Because of increased pulmonary blood flow.

Elevated cardiac output (CO) can lead to the development of pulmonary HTN.

Reason: Due to increased pulmonary arterial pressures.

Elevated left atrial pressure can lead to the development of pulmonary HTN.

Reason: Also due to increased pulmonary arterial pressures.

If a VSD is large and is not corrected, pulmonary arterial HTN may develop.

Reason: Pulmonary vascular obstruction develops.

Pregnancy can cause pulmonary HTN.

Reason: From increased pulmonary blood flow.

Pulmonary HTN can result from bronchiectasis.

Reasons: Due to an absolute loss of pulmonary cross-sectional area, along with acidosis, alveolar hypoxia, and polycythemia.

Pulmonary HTN can result from chronic thromboembolic disease.

Reason: Because of occlusion or narrowing of large to medium-sized arteries resulting in increased resistance to blood flow.

Pulmonary HTN can result from emphysema.

Reasons: Due to an absolute loss of pulmonary cross-sectional area, along with acidosis, alveolar hypoxia, and polycythemia.

Pulmonary HTN can result from obesity-hypoventilation syndrome.

Reasons: Because of alveolar hypoxia and arterial hypoxemia.

Pulmonary HTN can result from primary pulmonary artery tumors.

Reason: Due to occlusion or narrowing of large-sized to medium-sized arteries resulting in increased resistance to blood flow.

Pulmonary HTN and cor pulmonale occur with cystic fibrosis.

Reason: From chronic hypoxia.

Thyrotoxicosis can cause pulmonary HTN.

Reason: Because of increased pulmonary blood flow.

Pulmonary HTN can result from Takayasu's arteritis.

Reason: Due to occlusion or narrowing of large-sized to medium-sized arteries resulting in increased resistance to blood flow.

Blood Pressure (BP) -- Hypertension (HTN), Pulmonary – Signs and Symptoms

Hemoptysis may occur with mitral stenosis and mitral regurgitation.

Reason: Because of persistent pulmonary HTN.

Right axis deviation in an electrocardiogram (EKG) may occur with mitral stenosis.

Reason: Due to pulmonary HTN.

Syncope may occur with exertion in persons with severe primary pulmonary HTN.

Reason: The right ventricle is unable to provide appropriate CO to overcome the presence of obstruction or increased vascular resistance.

Blood Pressure (BP) -- Hypertension (HTN), Pulmonary – Treatment/ Management

Nitroglycerin may also relieve chest pain due to pulmonary HTN.

Reason: Nitroglycerin works primarily by relaxing smooth muscles.

Oxygen therapy may be administered to treat pulmonary HTN.

Reason: To reduce hypoxic pulmonary vasoconstriction.

Diuretic therapy may be administered to treat pulmonary HTN.

Reason: Reduction of fluid volume overload and venous congestion.

Diuretics are used with caution in patients with chronic obstructive pulmonary disease (COPD) who also have pulmonary HTN and cor pulmonale.

Reasons: (1) Diuretics are poorly tolerated in patients who are dependent upon preload and (2) Diuretics may precipitate metabolic alkalosis in hypercapnic patients.

Anticoagulation therapy may be administered to treat pulmonary HTN.

Reason: To reduce the likelihood of venous thrombus formation.

Blood Pressure (BP) -- Hypertension (HTN) – Rebound

Rebound HTN may occur if beta-blocker use is abruptly ended.

Reason: Probably due to up-regulation of beta-receptors.

Blood Pressure (BP) -- Hypertension (HTN) – Risk Factors

Aging increases the risk of developing HTN.

Reason: With age, there is stiffening of systemic arteries so that systolic pressure increases while diastolic pressure decreases.

Smokeless tobacco has been associated with HTN.

Reason: Probably due to its high sodium content.

Hypertension (HTN) and tachycardia occur with hyperthyroidism.

Reason: Heart rate increases to deliver oxygen and remove carbon dioxide from cells with increased rates of metabolism.

Sodium retention results in elevated BP.

Reasons: Sodium attracts water causing water retention. Water retention results in increased extracellular volume.

Sleep apnea can lead to systemic HTN.

Reason: Due to systemic vasoconstriction arising from decreased oxygen, increased carbon dioxide, and lowered pH.

With renal artery stenosis, HTN is associated with increased CO and systemic resistance.

Reasons: Because of (1) vasoconstriction from angiotensin II; (2) increased renal sodium and water retention because of angiotensin II and aldosterone; (3) increased blood volume which augments CO; and (4) promotion of cardiac and vascular hypertrophy from chronic elevation of angiotensin II.

Blood Pressure (BP) -- Hypertension (HTN) (HTN) – Secondary

Although secondary HTN accounts for less than 5% of HTN, a higher prevalence rate is noted for secondary HTN than primary (essential) HTN at specialized HTN clinics.

> Reason: Secondary HTN is more likely to be drug-resistant than primary (essential) HTN.

Up to 30% of patients referred to specialized HTN clinics have renovascular HTN, a common form of potentially curable secondary HTN.

> Reasons: Patients with HTN are often prescribed multiple antihypertensive drugs but renovascular HTN is often resistant to multiple drug antihypertensive regimens.

Secondary HTN occurs with acromegaly.

> Reason: Excess human growth hormone causes increased peripheral resistance.

Secondary HTN occurs with hypothyroidism.

> Reason: Mucopolysaccaride deposits in vascular tissues cause increased resistance.

Secondary HTN occurs with hypercalcemia.

Reasons: Elevated serum calcium levels cause increased vascular tone and increased peripheral resistance.

Blood Pressure (BP) -- Hypertension (HTN) – Signs and Symptoms

Assess the skin of hypertensive patients for cafe-au-lait spots.

Reason: Cafe-au-lait spots are an indication of neurofibromatosis.

The diagnosis of HTN is not based on a single BP reading.

Reason: One BP reading may not reflect the usual condition of the patient; as such, three or more occasions/ BP readings must be used before diagnosing HTN.

Blood Pressure (BP) -- Hypertension (HTN) – Transient

Transient HTN can develop in patients with second- or third-degree burns.

Reasons: Because of high circulating levels of catecholamines, renin, and angiotensin II.

Blood Pressure (BP) -- Hypertension (HTN) -- Treatment

Acute reduction of BP in a hypertensive individual can be detrimental.

> Reason: Reduction in BP, which is too great or too sudden, decreases the body's ability to autoregulate cerebral blood flow.

Beta-blockers should be used with extreme caution when treating HTN in patients with diabetes.

> Reasons: Beta-blockers may cause (1) blockade of hypoglycemic responses, (2) decrease in lipid levels and (3) impotence.

Beta-blockers may be administered to hypertensive persons who have excessive sympathetic stimulation from emotional stress.

> Reason: Beta-blockers inhibit the sympathetic-mediated release of renin.

Calcium channel blockers may be administered to persons with HTN and abnormal kidney function.

> Reason: Calcium channel blockers decrease vascular resistance by dilating the arterioles (resistance vessels).

Thiazide diuretics should be used with extreme caution when treating HTN in patients with diabetes.

> Reasons: Because of (1) worsened glucose levels and (2) worsened lipid profiles.

Regular aerobic exercise is included in the treatment regimen for HTN.

> Reasons: Regular aerobic exercise reduces arterial pressure and improves vascular function.

Hypertensive persons, being treated with a diuretic, may be concurrently treated with an angiotensin-converting enzyme (ACE) inhibitor or angiotensin receptor blocker (ARB).

> Reason: To prevent the renin-angiotensin-aldosterone system from being activated because of decreasing blood volume from the diuretic.

Most hypertensive patients are given a diuretic to stimulate renal secretion of sodium and water.

> Reasons: To reduce blood volume and arterial pressure.

Sodium restriction is included in the intervention for HTN.

> Reason: It may prevent progression of, or even reverse, cardiovascular changes that are associated with HTN.

Angiotensin-converting enzyme (ACE) inhibitors reduce BP.

Reason: They block the angiotensin converting enzyme responsible for cleaving angiotensin I to angiotensin II (a potent vasoconstrictor).

Patients with diabetes and HTN are particularly challenging to treat.

Reason: Many agents that lower BP may also adversely affect glucose metabolism.

Propranolol may be administered to a patient with Gullain-Barré syndrome.

Reason: To prevent tachycardia and HTN.

Clonidine may be administered to treat HTN complicated by renal disease.

Reason: Clonidine does not decrease renal blood flow or glomerular filtration.

Blood Pressure (BP) -- Hypertensive Emergency – In General and Physiology

Hypertensive emergency addresses malignant or accelerated HTN.

Reason: It turned out that malignant and accelerated HTN cover the same problem, and they were being used interchangeably.

Excess production of aldosterone can cause hypertensive emergency.

Reason: Due to the rapid rise in vascular resistance.

Excess production of angiotensin II can cause hypertensive emergency.

Reason: Also due to the rapid rise in vascular resistance.

Excess production of catecholamines can cause hypertensive emergency.

Reason: Because of the rapid rise in vascular resistance.

Excess production of endothelin can cause hypertensive emergency.

Reason: Also because of the rapid rise in vascular resistance.

Excess production of thromboxane can cause hypertensive emergency.

Reason: From the rapid rise in vascular resistance.

Excess production of vasopressin can cause hypertensive emergency.

Reason: Also from the rapid rise in vascular resistance.

Angiotensin II is directly cytotoxic to the blood vessel wall.

Reason: By activating gene expression for proinflammatory cytokines and transcription nuclear factor.

End-organ ischemia occurs with hypertensive emergency.

Reason: Due to compromised autoregulatory function.

Additional vasoactive substances are released in hypertensive emergencies.

Reason: In response to end-organ ischemia.

Deficient production of nitric oxide can cause hypertensive emergency.

Reason: Due to increased vasoreactivity.

Deficient production of prostacyclin can cause hypertensive emergency.

Reason: Also due to increased vasoreactivity.

While hypertensive emergency is more prevalent in patients with secondary HTN, essential HTN is more commonly the cause of hypertensive emergency.

> Reason: More people have essential HTN than secondary HTN.

Blood Pressure (BP) -- Hypertensive Emergency -- Types

Acute left ventricular dysfunction with pulmonary edema is a hypertensive emergency.

> Reason: Because of the possibility of impending or progressive target-organ dysfunction.

Acute myocardial infarction (MI) is a hypertensive emergency.

> Reason: Also due to the possibility of impending or progressive target-organ dysfunction.

Dissecting aortic aneurysm is a hypertensive emergency.

> Reason: Because of the possibility of impending or progressive target-organ dysfunction.

Eclampsia is a hypertensive emergency.

> Reason: Also due to the possibility of impending or progressive target-organ dysfunction.

Hypertensive encephalopathy is a hypertensive emergency.

Reason: Because of the possibility of impending or progressive target-organ dysfunction.

Intracerebral hemorrhage is a hypertensive emergency.

Reason: Also due to the possibility of impending or progressive target-organ dysfunction.

Unstable angina pectoris is a hypertensive emergency.

Reason: Because of the possibility of impending or progressive target-organ dysfunction.

Blood Pressure (BP) -- Hypertensive Emergency – Signs and Symptoms

Diagnosing hypertensive emergency solely on presenting symptoms can be difficult.

Reason: Most cases of hypertensive emergency are asymptomatic.

Back pain and chest pain in a hypertensive patient may suggest a hypertensive emergency.

Reason: These symptoms in a hypertensive patient may suggest possible aortic dissection.

Chest pain in a hypertensive patient may suggest a hypertensive emergency.

Reason: Chest pain in a hypertensive patient may suggest possible myocardial ischemia.

Shortness of breath (SOB) in a hypertensive patient may suggest a hypertensive emergency.

Reason: Shortness of breath (SOB) in a hypertensive patient may suggest possible pulmonary edema.

Headache and neck stiffness in a hypertensive patient may suggest a hypertensive emergency.

Reason: Headache and neck stiffness in a hypertensive patient may suggest a possible subarachnoid hemorrhage.

Headache, vomiting, confusion, and seizures in a hypertensive patient may suggest a hypertensive emergency.

Reason: Headache, vomiting, confusion, and seizures in a hypertensive patient may suggest possible hypertensive encephalopathy.

Blood Pressure (BP) -- Hypotension – Causes

Decreased BP occurs with cardiogenic shock.

Reasons: From (1) decreased CO and (2) decreased ejection fraction.

Low BP may occur with esophageal varices.

Reason: Due to blood loss.

Decreased CO and hypotension occur with tension pneumothorax.

Reason: Because of decreased venous return.

Cardiovascular signs and symptoms, including hypervolemia and hypotension, occur with uremia.

Reason: These signs and symptoms occur secondary to shifts of fluid into the extracellular space.

Hypotension may ensue if a grafted kidney is functioning well after renal transplantation.

Reason: Because of diuresis.

Hypotension and peripheral vasoconstriction with cold extremities may occur with adult respiratory distress syndrome (ARDS), also known as acute respiratory distress syndrome.

Reason: Adult or acute respiratory distress syndrome often occurs in the context of sepsis.

Hypotension can result from hypovolemia due to blood loss.

Reason: Decreased preload.

Septic shock (or Systemic Inflammatory Response Syndrome, SIRS) can cause hypotension.

Reason: Loss of vascular tone results from the release of bacterial endotoxins which activate the inflammatory cascade. The products of the inflammatory cascade include cytokines and nitric acid which cause systemic vasodilation.

Hypotension occurs with septic shock.

Reason: Initially from systemic vasodilation and later from cardiac depression.

Hypotension is a red flag (suggesting life-threatening condition) in individuals with chest pain.

Reason: The hypotension, in individuals with chest pain, is suggestive of decreased CO, possibly because of a large anterior MI.

Hypotension is common in heatstroke.

Reasons: (1) Vasodilation of cutaneous vessels, (2) pooling of blood in the venous system, (3) dehydration, and (4) myocardial damage.

The physical findings of hypotension, pulmonary edema and cyanosis are red flags for individuals with leg pain and swelling.

Reason: Hypotension, pulmonary edema and cyanosis suggest possible diagnosis of pulmonary embolism or HF or dysrhythmia.

Hypotension may occur during dialysis.

Reason: Most commonly from intravascular volume depletion.

Septic shock is usually characterized primarily by hypotension.

Reason: Due to decreased vascular tone.

Inadequate or impaired tissue perfusion occurs with neurogenic shock.

Reason: Because of decreased CO and BP.

Hematologic dysfunction occurs in shock.

Reasons: From hypotension, hypoxemia, acidosis, and stasis of capillary blood flow.

Caution must be exercised when rewarming an individual with myxedema coma. Do not do it too quickly.

Reason: Further vasodilation may occur, causing hypotension and shock.

Hypotension occurs with DKA.

Reason: Because of decreased renal blood flow.

Blood Pressure (BP) -- Hypotension – Consequences

Decreased tissue perfusion occurs with hypovolemic shock.

Reasons: From (1) decreased CO and (2) decreased systemic and pulmonic pressures.

Even though hypotension often occurs with cardiogenic shock, BP can be normal.

Reason: A significant increase in systemic resistance can occur with low flow states; as such, BP may appear to be normal.

Supine hypotension decreases uteroplacental blood flow.

Reason: Due to decreased maternal CO.

Syncope results from sudden impairment of brain metabolism.

Reason: Syncope usually results from hypotension with reduced cerebral blood flow.

Hypotension leads to tissue hypoxia.

Reasons: Because of reduced blood flow via decreased perfusion pressure and baroreceptor-mediated sympathetic activation (causing constriction of resistance vessels).

The reduced blood flow to organs, due to hypotension, is self-limiting.

Reason: The organs accumulate vasodilator metabolites which act to override the sympathetic-mediated vasoconstriction.

Arterial pressure decreases as hypotension progresses.

Reason: Metabolic acidosis impairs cardiac and vascular smooth muscle contraction, decreasing both CO and systemic vascular resistance.

Depression of all autonomic centers occurs as hypotension progresses.

Reason: The cardiovascular regulatory centers cease functioning.

The cardiovascular regulatory centers cease functioning as hypotension progresses.

Reason: Because of lack of oxygen.

The viscosity of the blood increases with hypotension.

Reasons: In the microcirculation, because of the low-flow state, (1) red blood cells adhere to each other, (2) leukocyte-endothelial adhesion is enhanced, and (3) platelet to platelet adhesion occurs.

Dehydration and hypotension cause further metabolic acidosis.

Reason: Due to impaired renal excretion of inorganic acids.

Hypotension can result from postintubation hyperinflation.

Reason: Decreased preload to the right ventricle.

Somatic death usually follows brain death within several days.

Reason: Because of progressive hypotension that becomes increasingly unresponsive to catecholamines.

Blood Pressure (BP) -- Hypotension – Medication Induced

Paralyzing agents may cause hypotension.

Reasons: From increased vagal stimulation and release of histamine; also because of ganglionic blockade.

Conduction delays, diminished CO and hypotension can result from calcium channel blockers.

Reason: Calcium is required for cellular contraction.

Barbiturates may cause hypotension and tachycardia.

Reason: They weaken the cardiovascular system.

Antidysrhythmics may cause hypotension.

Reason: Vasodilation causes decreased CO.

Local anesthetics may cause hypotension.

Reason: They weaken the cardiovascular system.

Blood Pressure (BP) -- Hypotension – Signs and Symptoms

Sedatives/ hypnotics may cause dizziness.

Reason: Because of hypotension.

Hypotension with abdominal pain is an ominous sign.

Reasons: Hypotension with abdominal pain suggests impending hemorrhagic, hypovolemic, or septic shock.

Blood Pressure (BP) -- Hypotension – Therapeutic Interventions

Volume resuscitation is important in a patient with increased intracranial pressure (ICP).

Reason: Hypotension is an important risk factor in increased ICP; it decreases cerebral perfusion pressure (CPP).

Pressor agents may be administered in the treatment of hypotension.

Reasons: Pressor agents increase arterial pressure by increasing systemic vascular resistance or stimulation of cardiac function.

Medications that stimulate the heart and dilate arterial vessels are used in the treatment of hypotension.

Reasons: Medications that stimulate the heart and dilate arterial vessels (1) improve cardiac function (by enhancing inotropy) and (2) decrease afterload on the heart.

If hypotension is severe, systemic vasodilators cannot be used alone.

Reason: Arterial pressure may fall more if systemic vasodilators are used alone.

Morphine may be contraindicated in volume-depleted persons.

Reason: Morphine may induce hypotension in volume-depleted persons.

Elevated arterial pressure is reduced slowly when treating preeclampsia.

Reasons: To avoid hypotension and decreased blood flow to the fetus.

Individuals with orthostatic hypotension should contract their calf muscles when standing for any time.

Reason: To increase venous blood flow.

Blood Pressure (BP) -- Hypotension Syndrome

Supine hypotensive syndrome can occur particularly during the third trimester of pregnancy.

Reason: Compression of the inferior vena cava diminishes venous return; thus, reducing CO and arterial pressure.

Blood Pressure (BP) -- Hypotension vs. Shock

Hypotension and shock are not the same thing.

Reason: Hypotension only becomes shock when inadequate tissue perfusion occurs (when blood pressure is inadequate for perfusion of the brain, heart, and kidneys).

Blood Pressure (BP) -- Hypotensive Shock

Hypotensive shock can progress to irreversible shock and death.

Reasons: Irreversible shock and death can occur from (1) cardiac depression, (2) sympathetic escape, (3) metabolic acidosis, (4) cerebral ischemia, and (5) systemic inflammatory responses.

Blood Pressure (BP) – Increased

The Valsalva maneuver and forceful sneezing are contraindicated in patients with cerebral aneurysm.

Reason: They can increase BP or obstruct venous return.

Increased BP occurs with stress.

Reason: Increased contraction of arteriolar smooth muscle because of norepinephrine release from the peripheral nerve endings.

Blood Pressure (BP) -- Intracranial Hypertension (HTN)

Visual changes may occur with brain tumors.

Reasons: The visual changes are caused by papilledema; chronic intracranial HTN causes the papilledema.

Anticonvulsant agents are administered prophylactically to patients with increased ICP.

Reason: To prevent seizures which cause the BP to increase.

Blood Pressure (BP) -- Medications Decreasing

Diuretics cause lowering of BP.

Reason: Reduction of effective plasma circulating volume lowers BP.

Blood Pressure (BP) -- Medications Increasing

Ephedrine raises both systolic and diastolic BPs.

Reasons: Ephedrine causes vasoconstriction and cardiac stimulation.

Oral adrenergic agents may raise the BP when they are used in doses sufficient to relieve nasal congestion.

Reason: Oral adrenergic agents are not selective.

In patients with inferior wall MI, nitroglycerin can cause HTN.

Reason: Persons with inferior wall MI are very sensitive to changes in preload.

Antidiuretic hormone (ADH) replacement is administered cautiously to patients with history of cardiac disease.

Reasons: Vasopressin (antidiuretic hormone, ADH) may cause HTN and overhydration.

Sympathomimetic-containing antihistamines are contraindicated in patients with HTN.

Reason: Sympathomimetic-containing antihistamines can elevate BP.

Orally administered estrogen can elevate BP.

Reason: First pass metabolism of orally administered estrogen in the liver produces angiotensinogen; the angiotensinogen elevates BP.

Ingestion of foods high in tyramine is contraindicated when taking monoamine oxidase inhibitors (MAOIs).

Reasons: Elevation of neurohormonal levels may cause (1) hypertensive crisis with vascular rupture, (2) cardiac dysrhythmia and (3) photophobia.

Corticosteroids are contraindicated in patients with HTN.

Reason: Corticosteroids elevate the BP.

Blood Pressure (BP) -- Medullary Hypertension (HTN)

The joint pain of osteoarthritis (OA) can arise from the subchondral bone.

Reason: Because of medullary HTN and/or microfractures in the subchondral bone.

Blood Pressure (BP) -- Near-Normal

The risk of stroke at near-normal BPs increases with preeclampsia.

> Reason: Due to abnormalities of cerebral circulatory autoregulation.

Blood Pressure (BP) – Orthopnea

Elevated intravascular pressure behind a failing pressure leads to orthopnea.

> Reason: Abnormal fluid accumulation.

Blood Pressure (BP) -- Orthostatic Hypotension

Orthostatic hypotension can occur after standing.

> Reasons: Due to blood pooling in the veins of the pelvis and the lower extremities leading to a significant reduction of venous return and stroke volume. If standing is prolonged, blood also extravasates in the extravascular space so that venous return is further reduced.

Normally, orthostatic hypotension is avoided with standing.

Reasons: Because of a reflex increase of sympathetic tone, peripheral and splanchnic vasoconstriction concurrent with increased heart rate. As such, even though CO may be reduced, BP is maintained.

A compensatory increase in either vascular resistance or heart rate with orthostasis may not occur with orthostatic hypotension.

Reason: As a consequence of autonomic failure.

Significant hypovolemia may cause orthostatic hypotension.

Reason: Sympathetic mechanisms may be inadequate to compensate for decreased venous return.

Decreased ability for vasoconstriction with position change leading to orthostatic hypotension may occur in the older patient.

Reasons: Because of (1) increased stiffness of peripheral vasculature and (2) decreased ability to adjust to changes in blood volume.

Diabetes increases the risk for orthostatic hypotension.

Reason: Due to autonomic dysfunction.

Older age increases the risk for orthostatic hypotension.

Reason: Also due to autonomic dysfunction.

Parkinson's disease increases the risk for orthostatic hypotension.

Reason: Because of autonomic dysfunction.

Orthostatic hypotension may occur with renal failure.

Reason: Volume depletion of venous circulation results in insufficient preload.

Postural drop of blood pressure may occur with esophageal varices.

Reason: Esophageal varices cause blood loss; the postural drop of BP may occur because of the blood loss.

Drugs can cause orthostatic hypotension.

Reasons: By causing volume depletion or vasodilation. Note: The following drugs can cause orthostatic hypotension: adrenergic neuron blocking drugs, alcohol, alpha-adrenergic blocking drugs, angiotensin-converting enzyme inhibitors, antidepressants, diuretics, centrally acting hypotensive drugs, ganglion blocking drugs, tranquilizers, and vasodilators.

Multiple system atrophy (Shy-Drager syndrome) can cause orthostatic hypotension.

Reason: Due to being a primary disorder of autonomic failures. Note: Other primary disorders of autonomic failures include Parkinson's disease with autonomic failure and pure autonomic failure (Bradbury-Eggleston syndrome).

A patient taking Enalapril maleate (Vasotec) should change position slowly.

Reason: To reduce orthostatic hypotension.

Antihypertensives may cause dizziness.

Reason: Because of orthostatic hypotension.

Orthostatic hypotension can result from prolonged bed rest.

Reason: Circulating blood volume decreases during prolonged bed rest.

Some patients with orthostatic hypotension also experience HTN when supine.

Reason: Inability to regulate vascular tone because of severe autonomic dysfunction or severely non-compliant arteries.

The mechanisms of syncope that follows within 1 hour post-prandially are similar to those for orthostatic hypotension.

> Reasons: Peripheral vasodilation and splanchnic blood pooling develop due to digestion.

Blood Pressure (BP) -- Physiologic Maintenance of

Increased peripheral vascular resistance occurs with hypothyroidism.

> Reason: The increased peripheral vascular resistance is an attempt to maintain systolic BP with a lowered CO.

The kidney provides for long-term control of BP.

> Reasons: The kidney alters blood volume; BP changes with blood volume.

Increased potassium intake can decrease BP.

> Reasons: (1) Production and release of renin are suppressed; (2) natriuresis is induced and (3) tension in blood vessel walls is decreased.

Blood Pressure (BP) -- Postural Orthostatic Tachycardia Syndrome (POTS)

In cases of postural orthostatic tachycardia syndrome (POTS), peripheral vascular resistance does not increase in response to orthostatic stress.

Reason: Due to autonomic dysfunction.

Blood pressure is still maintained with POTS.

Reason: Because of increased heart rate.

Cardiac output is still maintained with POTS.

Reason: Also due to increased heart rate.

Near-syncope develops in individuals with POTS.

Reason: Likely due to flow maldistribution and cerebral flow reduction.

Severe fatigue develops in individuals with POTS.

Reason: Also likely due to flow maldistribution and cerebral flow reduction.

Excessive tachycardia occurs with POTS.

Reason: As a consequence of orthostasis and over activation of the sympathetic system.

Blood Pressure (BP) -- Portal Hypertension (HTN)

Vasocongestion within the intestinal vasculature (from portal HTN) can lead to ascites.

Reason: Plasma transudates into the abdominal cavity.

Portal HTN can lead to redistribution of blood flow (reduced renal perfusion).

Reason: Because of the persistence of amine neurotransmitters.

Portal HTN can cause congestive splenomegaly.

Reason: The splenic vein drains into the portal vein.

Portal HTN can lead to increased production of aldosterone.

Reason: Due to redistribution of blood flow (reduced renal perfusion).

Portal HTN can lead to persistence of amine neurotransmitters.

Reason: Development of collateral venous vessels.

Portal HTN can lead to transudation of plasma into the abdominal cavity.

Reason: Because of vasocongestion within the intestinal vasculature.

Portal HTN can lead to increased sodium and water retention.

Reason: Increased production of aldosterone.

Portal HTN can lead to dilation of lymph channels draining the liver.

Reason: Increased production of liver lymph (high protein).

A dramatic increase in portal vascular resistance (portal HTN) occurs with liver disease.

Reason: Due to decreased portal vascular radius.

Blood Pressure (BP) -- Pulmonary Arterial HTN (PAH)

Pulmonary arterial HTN (PAH) is not the only cause of pulmonary HTN (PH).

Reasons: Pulmonary HTN (PH) can also develop as a result of, but not restricted to, hypoxemic lung disorders (e.g., alveolar hypoventilation disorders, chronic exposure to high altitudes, chronic obstructive pulmonary disease (COPD), developmental lung disorders, interstitial lung disease, sleep-disordered breathing), left heart disease [such as left ventricular diastolic dysfunction, left ventricular systolic dysfunction, valvular disease], hematologic disorders [such as chronic hemolytic anemia, myeloproliferative disorders], metabolic disorders [such as Gaucher disease, glycogen storage disease, thyroid disorders],systemic disorders [such as lymphangioleiomyomatosis, pulmonary histiocytosis, sarcoidosis], or thromboembolism (or chronic thromboembolic pulmonary HTN or CTEPH).

In normal healthy individuals, pulmonary arterial pressure (PAP) increases only slightly with increased CO.

Reason: Due to the compensatory increase of the cross-sectional area of the pulmonary vascular bed.

Pulmonary arterial smooth muscle cell hypertrophy develops with PAH.

Reasons: As a consequence of the elevated pulmonary arterial pressure and sustained vasoconstriction which occur with PAH.

Dilation of the vessel lumen may develop with PAH.

Reason: Due to marked hypertrophy of the pulmonary arterial smooth muscle.

Fibrosis may develop with PAH.

Reason: Because of marked hypertrophy of the pulmonary arterial smooth muscle.

Medial atrophy may develop with PAH.

Reason: Marked hypertrophy of the pulmonary arterial smooth muscle.

The right heart has to overcome increased afterload with PAH.

Reason: As a consequence of increased resistance to circulatory flow.

Functional decline of right heart develops with PAH.

Reason: As a consequence of progressive and inexorable HF.

Death ultimately results from untreated PAH.

Reason: As a consequence of functional decline of the right heart.

If a VSD is large and is not corrected, PAH may develop.

Reason: Development of pulmonary vascular obstruction.

Fixed PAH develops with mitral valve stenosis.

Reasons: From (1) hypertrophy of the media and (2) intimal thickening of the pulmonary arterioles.

Pulmonary artery HTN (PAH) may occur with VSD.

Reason: From long-term pulmonary overcirculation or overload.

Blood Pressure (BP) -- Pulmonary HTN (PH)

Syncope may occur with exertion in patients with severe primary PH.

Reason: The right ventricle is unable to provide appropriate CO to overcome the presence of obstruction or increased vascular resistance.

Oxygen therapy may be administered to treat PH.

Reason: To reduce hypoxic pulmonary vasoconstriction.

Right axis deviation in an electrocardiogram (EKG) may occur with mitral stenosis.

Reason: Due to PH.

Hemoptysis may occur with mitral regurgitation.

Reason: Because of PH.

Sleep apnea can lead to left heart failure.

Reasons: (1) Decreased pleural pressure and increased cardiac afterload arising from decreased oxygen, increased carbon dioxide, and lowered pH; and (2) PH and right heart failure arising from decreased oxygen, increased carbon dioxide, and lowered pH.

Right-sided HF may occur late with chronic mitral insufficiency.

Reason: Increased pulmonary pressures.

Blood Pressure (BP) -- Pulmonary HTN (PH) -- Signs and Symptoms/ Comorbidities

An accentuated pulmonary component of S2 may be audible at the apex of over 90% of patients with PH.

Reason: Likely due to high pulmonary pressure increasing the force of pulmonic valve closure.

Accessory muscle use may occur with PH.

Reason: Because of pulmonary parenchymal disease.

Arthritis may occur with PH.

Reason: Likely due to a connective tissue disorder.

Ascites may occur with PH.

Reason: Because of portal HTN.

Caput medusae may occur with PH.

Reason: Likely due to portal HTN.

Central cyanosis may occur with PH.

Reasons: Because of an abnormal V/Q intrapulmonary shunt, hypoxemia, and pulmonary-to-systemic shunt.

Clubbing may occur with PH.

Reasons: Likely due to congenital heart disease and/or pulmonary venoocclusive disease.

Cool extremities may be present in someone with advanced PH with right ventricular failure.

Reason: Because of reduced CO.

Crackles may occur with PH.

Reasons: Likely due to (1) pulmonary congestion and/or effusion or (2) pulmonary parenchymal disease.

Decreased breath sounds may occur with PH.

Reason: Because of pulmonary congestion and/or effusion.

A diastolic murmur may occur with moderate-to-severe PH.

Reason: Likely due to pulmonary regurgitation.

Diminished pulse pressure may be present in someone with advanced PH with right ventricular failure.

Reason: Because of reduced CO.

Distention of jugular veins may be present in someone with advanced PH with right ventricular failure.

Reasons: Likely as a result of right ventricular dysfunction and/or tricuspid regurgitation.

Dull breath sounds may occur with PH.

Reasons: Because of pulmonary congestion and/or effusion.

Dyspnea on exertion may occur with PH.

Reason: Likely as a result of activation of stretch receptors in the pulmonary arteries and right ventricle.

An early systolic click may be present in someone with PH.

Reason: Because of the sudden interruption of the opening of the pulmonary valve into a high pressure artery.

Enlarged tonsils may occur with PH.

Reason: Likely due to disordered ventilation and sleep apnea.

Hemoptysis may occur with mitral regurgitation.

Reason: As a consequence of PH.

Hemoptysis may occur with mitral stenosis.

Reason: From persistent PH.

Hepatojugular reflux may occur with moderate-to-severe PH.

Reason: Likely due to high central venous pressure.

A holosystolic murmur (best auscultated in the fourth interspace to the left of the sternum) eventually develops as PH persists.

Reason: As a consequence of tricuspid insufficiency.

Icterus may occur with PH.

Reason: Likely due to portal HTN.

An increased jugular "a" wave may occur with PH.

Reason: Likely as a result of poor right ventricular compliance.

A left parasternal lift may be present in individuals with PH.

Reasons: Likely due to the presence of high ventricular pressure and hypertrophy.

Low BP may be present in patients with advanced PH with right ventricular failure.

Reason: Likely as a result of reduced CO.

Macroglossia may occur with PH.

Reasons: Likely due to disordered ventilation and sleep apnea.

A midsystolic ejection murmur may be present in patients with PH.

Reason: Likely as a result of turbulent transvalvular pulmonary outflow.

A narrowed pharyngeal opening may occur with PH.

Reasons: Likely due to disordered ventilation and sleep apnea.

Obesity may occur with PH.

Reasons: Also as a result of disordered ventilation and sleep apnea.

Palmar erythema may occur with PH.

Reason: Likely due to portal HTN.

A palpable cardiac impulse near the left sternal border and in the hypogastrium develops as PH persists.

Reason: Because of the enlargement of the right ventricle.

Peripheral cyanosis often develops late in the course of PH.

Reason: The peripheral cyanosis is secondary to reduced CO and peripheral vasoconstriction.

Peripheral venous insufficiency or obstruction may occur with PH.

Reason: Due to possible venous thrombosis.

A productive cough may occur with PH.

Reason: Likely because of pulmonary parenchymal disease.

Protracted expiration may occur with PH.

Reason: Also likely due to pulmonary parenchymal disease.

Pulmonary vascular bruits may occur with PH.

Reason: Likely from chronic thromboembolic PH.

Rash may occur with PH.

Reason: Likely because of a connective tissue disorder.

Raynaud's phenomenon may occur with PH.

Reason: Also likely from a connective tissue disorder.

A right ventricular S3 occurs in 23% of patients with advanced PH with right ventricular failure.

Reason: Likely due to right ventricular dysfunction.

A right ventricular S4 occurs in 38% of patients with PH.

Reasons: Likely because of the presence of high ventricular pressure (increased filling pressure) and hypertrophy of the right side of the heart.

A right-sided (ventricular) diastolic (S3) gallop, accentuated by inspiration, may develop as PH persists.

Reason: Due to cor pulmonale.

Sclerodactyly may occur with PH.

Reason: Likely because of a connective tissue disorder.

Spider angiomata may occur with PH.

Reason: Likely from portal HTN.

Splenomegaly may occur with PH.

Reason: Also likely due to portal HTN.

Syncope may occur with exertion in patients with severe primary PH.

Reason: The right ventricle is unable to provide appropriate CO to overcome the presence of obstruction or increased vascular resistance.

Substernal pain from PH may be misdiagnosed as classic angina pectoris.

Reason: Substernal pain from PH is often precipitated by exertion.

Telangiectasia may occur with PH.

Reason: Likely because of a connective tissue disorder.

Venous stasis ulcers may occur with PH.

Reason: Possibly from sickle cell disease.

Wheezing may occur with PH.

Reason: Likely due to pulmonary parenchymal disease.

Blood Pressure (BP) -- Pulmonary HTN (PH) – Diagnosis

Blood serologies (e.g., complete blood count (CBC), antinuclear antibodies (ANA), antiphospholipid antibodies, human immunodeficiency virus (HIV), liver function, and renal function) are included in the assessment of PH.

Reasons: To exclude various causes of PH including collagen vascular disease, infection, liver disease, and renal disease.

Computed tomography (CT) scan of the chest may be used as contingent tests of patients with PH.

Reasons: To assess adenopathy and interstitial lung disease.

Echocardiograms are used in the evaluation of possible PH.

Reason: To estimate pulmonary artery (PA) pressure, suggesting a left-sided etiology, and showing signs of PH severity.

Echocardiograms are, by themselves, inadequate to make a diagnosis of PH.

> Reason: About half of echocardiographic diagnoses of PH are false positive.

An echocardiogram is used in the detection of PH.

> Reasons: To evaluate heart chamber sizes and function, to assess valvular abnormalities, and to evaluate for the presence of PH.

An echocardiogram with a contrast bubble is used in the detection of PH.

> Reason: To evaluate possible shunt.

An electrocardiogram is used in the detection of PH.

> Reason: To exclude other causes of cardiopulmonary symptoms.

A lung (V/Q) scan is utilized in the assessment of PH.

> Reason: To exclude thromboembolism.

Overnight oximetry is utilized in the assessment of PH.

> Reason: To screen for sleep-disordered breathing.

An oxygen desaturation study may be utilized in the assessment of PH.

Reason: To evaluate the need for supplemental oxygen (at rest and during exertion).

A polysomnogram may be used as a contingent test of patients with PH.

Reasons: To help in the diagnosis and treatment of sleep-disordered breathing.

Pulmonary function testing (PFT) is used in the assessment of PH.

Reason: To exclude intrinsic lung disease.

Right cardiac catheterization may be used in the assessment of PH.

Reasons: To confirm the diagnosis of PH, to assess other cardiac causes (e.g., shunt), and to assist in the consideration of possible left heart catherization.

Catherization is used in the diagnosis of PH.

Reason: To confirm both the diagnosis and etiology of PH.

Catherization is used to assess pulmonary capillary wedge pressure (PCWP) of patients with suspected PH.

Reason: To determine if the PH is secondary to left HF.

A six-minute walk test may be used in the assessment of PH.

Reason: To establish a baseline of the patient's endurance.

A transesophageal echocardiogram may be used as a contingent test of patients with PH.

Reasons: To assess patent foramen ovale (PFO) and to characterize valvular function.

Blood Pressure (BP) – Pulmonary HTN (PH) – Management/ Treatment

Oxygen therapy may be administered to treat PH.

Reason: To reduce hypoxic pulmonary vasoconstriction.

Nitroglycerin may also relieve chest pain due to PH.

Reason: Nitroglycerin works primarily by relaxing smooth muscles.

Diuretic therapy may be administered to treat PH.

Reasons: To reduce fluid volume overload and venous congestion.

Diuretics are used with caution in patients with chronic obstructive pulmonary disease (COPD) who also have PH and cor pulmonale.

Reasons: (1) Diuretics are tolerated poorly in patients who are dependent on preload and (2) Diuretics may precipitate metabolic alkalosis in a hypercapnic patient.

Anticoagulation therapy may be administered to treat PH.

Reason: To reduce likelihood of venous thrombus formation.

Blood Pressure (BP) -- Pulse Pressure

A wide pulse pressure develops with aortic insufficiency.

Reason: From low aortic diastolic pressure and high systemic pressures.

Wide pulse pressure occurs with aortic regurgitation.

Reason: Due to runoff of blood back into the left ventricle.

Blood Pressure (BP) -- Renal Vascular HTN

Peripheral vascular resistance is increased as a result of renal vascular HTN.

> Reason: Decreased renal perfusion (from renal vascular HTN) stimulates renin release by the affected kidney.

Blood Pressure (BP) -- Secondary HTN

Secondary HTN occurs with acute stress.

> Reason: Release of catecholamines and glucocorticoids is precipitated by acute stress.

Fibromuscular dysplasia in young women can cause secondary HTN.

> Reason: Renal artery stenosis leads to decreased renal blood flow; the decreased blood flow then causes increased renin release and HTN.

Atherosclerosis in older patients can cause secondary HTN.

> Reasons: Also due to renal artery stenosis leading to decreased renal blood flow; the decreased blood flow then causes increased renin release and HTN.

Secondary HTN occurs with primary aldosteronism.

Reason: Excess aldosterone promotes sodium retention.

Secondary HTN occurs with cortical disturbances.

Reason: Glucocorticoids facilitate sodium and water retention.

Blood Pressure (BP) -- Standing

An abrupt drop in venous return to the heart occurs when an individual stands.

Reason: Due to 500 to 800 ml of blood being displaced to the abdomen and lower extremities when standing.

Decreased CO occurs when an individual stands.

Reason: Because of the abrupt drop in venous return to the heart.

A reflex increase in sympathetic outflow occurs on standing.

Reasons: From the stimulation of aortic, carotid, and cardiopulmonary baroreceptors.

Heart rate, cardiac contractility and vascular resistance normally increase on standing.

Reason: In order to maintain a stable systemic BP.

Toxins Changing Blood Pressure (BP)

Nicotine initially causes increased BP and cardiac rate.

Reasons: Neurotransmitters are released from both adrenergic terminals and the adrenal medulla.

Blood Pressure (BP) – Treatment/ Management

Vasopressors may be used in the treatment of neurogenic shock.

Reason: Vasopressors maintain BP and organ perfusion.

Beta-blockers reduce BP.

Reasons: Beta-blockers (1) decrease CO (primary reason); (2) decrease sympathetic outflow from the central nervous system (CNS); and (3) inhibit renin release from the kidneys.

Angiotensin-converting enzyme (ACE) inhibitors are used for treating HTN in patients with diabetes.

Reasons: Angiotensin-converting enzyme (ACE) inhibitors are glucose-neutral and lipid-neutral; thus, positively impacting the cardiovascular profile.

Chapter 3: Blood Supply, Blood Volume and Circulation

Blood Supply

Prolonged wound healing occurs with diabetes mellitus.

Reason: Impaired blood supply.

Gastric ulcers heal slowly.

Reason: Poor blood supply.

Blood Volume

Increased blood volume is a consequence of the stress syndrome.

Reasons: Because of (1) aldosterone effects (which increases sodium and water reabsorption/ retention), and

(2) antidiuresis from antidiuretic hormone (ADH) (causing decreased urine production and increased water retention).

Decreased ability for vasoconstriction with position change leading to orthostatic hypotension may occur in older patients.

Reasons: From (1) increased stiffness of peripheral vasculature and (2) decreased ability to adjust to changes in blood volume.

Hypertensive persons, being treated with a diuretic, may be concurrently treated with an angiotensin-converting enzyme (ACE) inhibitor or angiotensin receptor blocker (ARB).

Reason: To prevent the renin-angiotensin-aldosterone system from being activated because of decreased blood volume from the diuretic.

Most hypertensive patients are given a diuretic to stimulate renal secretion of sodium and water.

Reasons: To reduce blood volume and arterial pressure.

Adrenal adenoma can cause renal retention of sodium and water, increasing blood volume and arterial pressure.

Reason: Increased aldosterone secretion.

Adrenal hyperplasia can lead to renal retention of sodium and water, increasing blood volume and arterial pressure.

Reason: Also due to increased aldosterone secretion.

Renal retention of sodium and water are necessary to sustain a hypertensive state.

Reason: To increase blood volume.

In hypovolemic states, restoration of reduced blood volume increases CO (that had been reduced by hypovolemia).

Reason: The restoration of the reduced blood volume increases the preload on the heart.

Hyperthyroidism can lead to HTN.

Reasons: Because of (1) induction of systemic vasoconstriction, (2) increased blood volume and (3) increased cardiac activity.

Hypertension (HTN) and volume expansion occur in Cushing's syndrome.

Reason: From excessive glucocorticoids.

Blood volume, CO, and arterial pressure increase in hypertensive patients.

Reason: Altered renal function leads to sodium and water retention.

With aortic stenosis, the distal pressures are not as low as one would expect from hemodynamics alone.

> Reasons: Reduced systemic blood flow (renal blood flow in particular) causes increased renin release and activation of the renin-angiotensin-aldosterone system; elevated blood volume and arterial pressure result.

Orthostatic hypotension can result from prolonged bed rest.

> Reason: Decreased circulating blood volume.

Impaired blood flow occurs with polycythemia.

> Reasons: Because of hypervolemia and hyperviscosity of the blood.

Preload is increased during pregnancy.

> Reason: Increased blood volume.

Increased metabolic acidosis occurs in a patient with diabetic ketoacidosis who is also suffering from diminished vascular volume.

> Reason: Diminished tissue perfusion.

With septic shock, the amount of oxygen delivered to the cells decreases.

> Reason: Maldistribution of circulating blood volume.

Interference in venous return may lead to reduced CO.

Reason: About three-fourths of the systemic blood volume is contained within the venous bed.

Prerenal azotemia results from renal hypoperfusion.

Reason: Decreased effective arterial blood volume.

Increased blood glucose occurs in patients with diabetic ketoacidosis (while vascular volume falls).

Reason: Decreased glomerular filtration.

Circulatory stasis occurs with polycythemia.

Reasons: Because of hypervolemia and hyperviscosity of the blood.

Blood vessel distention occurs with polycythemia.

Reasons: Also because of hypervolemia and hyperviscosity of the blood.

Decreased circulating volume occurs in anaphylactic shock.

Reasons: Due to peripheral vasodilation and increased capillary membrane permeability.

With polycythemia, blood circulation is impaired.

Reasons: From hypervolemia (increased volume) and hyperviscosity (increased viscosity) of the blood.

Fluid replacement is a priority for patients suffering from hemorrhage.

Reason: Loss of circulating blood volume results in deficiency of fluid volume and decline in CO.

Circulation -- Abdominal Compartment Syndrome

With abdominal compartment syndrome, ischemia and necrosis of tissues (and organs) occurs within the abdominal cavity.

Reason: Increased pressure within the abdominal cavity compromises circulation.

Circulation -- Circulatory Insufficiency

Metabolic acidosis is a possibility for patients suffering from hypothermia.

Reason: Because of circulatory insufficiency with increased metabolic activity (from shivering).

Circulation -- Circulatory Overload

Fluid restriction is essential when treating renal failure.

> Reason: To prevent circulatory overload and interstitial edema.

Circulation -- Collateral

Esophageal varices may occur with liver cirrhosis.

> Reason: Due to increased blood flow to the veins as collateral circulation develops in which blood from the intestines goes directly to the vena cava.

With esophageal varices, collateral circulation develops which diverts blood to the systemic veins.

> Reason: Response to increased venous pressure caused by the obstruction of portal venous flow which results in rise in portal venous pressure.

Women may have atypical symptoms of ischemia.

> Reasons: Women have smaller diameter coronary arteries and less developed collateral circulation.

Circulation -- Compromised

Patients with pelvic fractures who are hemodynamically unstable are at immediate risk of death.

> Reason: Because of compromised circulation.

Circulation -- Impaired

Gangrenous necrosis may occur in the lower legs of patients suffering from impaired circulation.

> Reasons: From severe hypoxia and subsequent ischemic injury.

Circulation -- Improving

An injured extremity should be elevated.

> Reasons: To (1) reduce edema, (2) increase venous return and blood circulation and (3) reduce pain.

Chapter 4: Peripheral Circulation, Peripheral Arterial Disease and Peripheral Vascular Disease

Chapter 4: Peripheral Circulation, Peripheral Arterial Disease and Peripheral Vascular Disease

Peripheral Circulation -- Acute Limb Ischemia

The viability of a limb is endangered with acute limb ischemia.

> Reason: As a consequence of sudden reduction of limb perfusion because of an acute interruption of blood flow. Note: Ischemia is considered to be acute when it presents within two weeks following an occlusive event.

Peripheral Circulation -- Age-Related Changes

Slowed circulation to the periphery is an age-related change.

> Reason: Because of rigid arteries.

Nail growth rate declines with aging.

Reason: From decreased peripheral circulation.

Peripheral Circulation -- Deep Vein/Venous Thrombosis (DVT)

Deep venous thrombosis (DVT) is a common complication of pregnancy.

Reasons: Pregnancy is characterized by a hypercoagulable state because of (1) venous stasis; (2) decreasing fibrinolytic activity; and (3) increased procoagulant factors.

Anticoagulation is a standard treatment for both DVT and pulmonary embolism.

Reason: Increased recurrence with delayed or inadequate anticoagulation.

Deep vein thrombosis (DVT) may occur with neurogenic shock.

Reason: From venous pooling in the lower extremities.

Aspirin is effective in preventing DVT.

Reason: Aspirin has anticoagulant effects caused by inhibition of prostaglandin production; prostaglandins cause platelets to aggregate and participate in the formation of clots.

Except in research settings, contrast venography is usually not done for patients with DVT.

Reason: Contrast venography is invasive and has potential complications.

Sequential compression stockings or intermittent plantar compression pumps may be applied prophylactically to both legs of injured persons.

Reason: To prevent DVT.

Peripheral Circulation -- Insufficient

Numbness and burning of toes occur with polycythemia vera.

Reason: Because of peripheral vascular insufficiency.

Numbness and burning of toes and feet occur with diabetes.

Reason: Also due to peripheral vascular insufficiency.

Peripheral Circulation -- Peripheral Artery/Arterial Disease (PAD) – Pathophysiology

Acute or critical ischemia can result from peripheral arterial disease (PAD).

> Reason: Due to systemic atherosclerosis leading to reduction of a limb's blood supply. Note: One or more territories of the aortoiliac, femoral-popliteal, and infra-popliteal arteries may be affected by PAD.

Both tissue ischemia and a pressure drop distal to the luminal obstruction occur in PAD.

> Reason: An atherosclerosis associated flow-limiting stenosis exists in the arterial system of the lower extremities.

Assuming that a subclavian stenosis does not exist, the systolic BP in the lower extremity is lower relative to the systolic BP in the upper extremity.

> Reason: A BP drop distal to the luminal obstruction may be occurring in the lower extremity.

Intermittent claudification (IC) and gangrene of the feet or toes are representative conditions of PAD.

> Reason: Tissue ischemia and necrosis (in the case of gangrene) result from an extensive accumulation of atherosclerotic plaques.

Revascularization cases -- to restore adequate oxygen supply to a region distal to an obstruction – are also classified as PAD.

> Reason: Because of the underlying cause of the arterial obstruction.

A severe PAD is frequently associated with advanced coronary artery disease and cerebrovascular disease.

> Reason: Systemic involvement of atherosclerosis.

Peripheral Circulation -- Peripheral Arterial Disease (PAD) – Signs and Symptoms

Symptoms of PAD are more common in the lower extremities than in the upper extremities.

> Reason: Because of higher incidence of obstructive lesions in the lower extremities.

Calf claudication (walking-induced pain) can occur because of PAD.

> Reason: Calf claudication is commonly a manifestation of superficial femoral artery disease.

Cramping, tightness, or tiredness may occur anywhere from the buttocks to the feet of someone with PAD.

Reason: As a consequence of arterial claudication.

Gluteal claudication (walking-induced pain) can occur because of PAD.

Reason: Gluteal claudication is commonly a manifestation of distal aortic disease.

Leg edema may develop in persons with PAD.

Reason: Individuals with PAD have to dangle the affected leg over the edge of the bed in order to sleep with less pain.

Pain from PAD may worsen when walking uphill.

Reason: Due to arterial claudication.

A reduction in femoral pulse does not always indicate PAD.

Reason: A reduction in femoral pulse can result from body habitus or a deep femoral artery.

Assess the dorsalis pedis pulse when evaluating patients for possible PAD.

Reason: A normal dorsalis pedis pulse rules out significant obstructive PAD with 92% accuracy.

Assess the posterior tibial pulse when evaluating patients for possible PAD.

Reason: A normal posterior tibial pulse rules out significant obstructive PAD with 96% accuracy.

Pain during rest, non-healing ulcerations, or gangrene may occur with PAD.

Reason: As a presentation of critical limb ischemia.

Thigh pain can occur because of PAD.

Reason: Commonly as a manifestation of iliac disease.

Ulcers and gangrenes may develop (predominately affecting the toes) in individuals with PAD.

Reason: Blood flow to the limb is insufficient to maintain cell viability at rest. Note: Ulcers and gangrenes can also occur in the ankle and heel.

Peripheral Circulation -- Peripheral Arterial Disease (PAD) – Assessment/Diagnosis

The diagnosis of PAD is more important than simply the associating it with lower extremity ischemia.

Reason: Patients with PAD have increased cardiovascular mortality (e.g., from MI, stroke).

Assess the amount of exercise necessary to elicit claudication symptoms.

Reason: The severity of stenosis and the amount of exercise necessary to elicit claudication symptoms are correlated.

Physical assessment addressing PAD involves checking the patient's lower extremities.

Reason: To assess for signs of acute or chronic peripheral ischemia.

Do not palpate the abdomen when performing a physical assessment addressing PAD.

Reason: This may cause rupture of an abdominal aortic aneurysm.

Confirm the diagnosis of PAD using noninvasive tests.

Reason: The prevalence of PAD is underestimated when the diagnosis is based on symptoms alone or on pulse palpation.

Peripheral Arterial Disease (PAD) – Assessment/ Diagnosis – Differential Diagnosis

When assessing for possible PAD, note for burning or tingling sensations (particularly in the hands and feet).

Reason: Peripheral neuropathy may be responsible.

When assessing for possible PAD, note for ischemia of the distal extremities especially in young smokers.

Reason: Buerger's disease may be responsible.

When assessing for possible PAD, note for muscle pain in the calves and feet.

Reason: Night cramps may be responsible.

When assessing for possible PAD, note for numbness and pain in the forefoot.

Reason: Neuroma may be responsible.

When assessing for possible PAD, note for pain and swelling in the small joints, particularly in the hands.

Reason: Rheumatoid arthritis (RA) may be responsible.

When assessing for possible PAD, note for pain, stiffness, and burning in the soles of the feet.

Reason: Plantar fasciitis may be responsible.

When assessing for possible PAD, note for pain, weakness, and loss of sensation in the posterior aspect of the lower limbs.

Reason: Nerve root compression may be responsible.

When assessing for possible PAD, note for severe pain in the joints of the feet, ankles, hands, and wrists.

Reason: Gout may be responsible.

Peripheral Circulation -- Peripheral Arterial Disease (PAD) – Management/ Treatment

Use of elastic hoses is contraindicated for individuals with PAD.

Reason: Elastic hoses reduce the blood flow to the skin and lower extremities.

Well-fitting and protective shoes are indicated for individuals with PAD.

Reason: To reduce trauma.

The use of moisturizing creams on the feet is indicated for individuals with PAD.

Reason: To protect against excessive drying.

A daily aspirin may be indicated for individuals with PAD.

Reasons: To lower the risk of cerebral vascular accident (CVA) and/ or MI.

Treatment of dyslipidemia is included in the management of PAD.

Reasons: To prevent claudication and reduce the progression of the disease.

Treatment of HTN is included in the management of PAD.

Reasons: Hypertension (HTN) is not only a risk factor for PAD but HTN also increases the risk for developing symptoms of PAD.

Arterial revascularization may be performed distal to an obstruction, if present in a PAD.

Reasons: To restore adequate oxygen supply to the distal extremities and to avoid amputation.

Cessation of smoking is an important component in management of PAD.

Reasons: Nicotine in cigarette smoke causes vasoconstriction. Cessation of smoking reduces amputation risk by10-fold and mortality risk by 50%.

Individuals with critical limb ischemia need to be promptly referred to a hospital with a vascular surgery team.

> Reason: The limb's blood supply must be reestablished immediately to prevent imminent risk of limb loss.

Peripheral Circulation -- Perfusion

The skin of a person hemorrhaging may be cool and moist.

> Reason: From poor peripheral perfusion.

Peripheral Circulation -- Peripheral Embolism

Even though anticoagulants do not improve the prognosis of patients after an MI, they are administered in the early discharge phase.

> Reason: To promote reduction of peripheral embolization.

Peripheral Circulation -- Peripheral Vascular Disease (PVD)

Peripheral vascular disease (PVD) is different from peripheral arterial disease (PAD).

> Reasons: Peripheral vascular disease (PVD) includes disorders of both the venous and arterial systems, while peripheral arterial disease (PAD) is atherosclerosis of the lower extremity arterial system.

Peripheral vascular disease occurs in patients with diabetes.

> Reason: Diabetes accelerates macrovascular disease.

Peripheral Circulation -- Peripheral Vascular Resistance

Angina is more likely to occur during exposure to cold.

> Reason: Increased peripheral vascular resistance results in increased myocardial work.

Increased peripheral vascular resistance occurs with hypothyroidism.

> Reason: The increased peripheral vascular resistance is an attempt to maintain the systolic BP with a lowered CO.

Decreased ability for vasoconstriction with position change leading to orthostatic hypotension may occur in older patients.

Reasons: From (1) increased stiffness of peripheral vasculature and (2) decreased ability to adjust to changes in blood volume.

Increased regurgitant flow, along with raised diastolic filling pressure and volume, occur in chronic aortic insufficiency.

Reason: Because of increased peripheral resistance (e.g., in HTN).

Secondary HTN occurs with hypercalcemia.

Reasons: Increased vascular tone and peripheral resistance caused by elevated serum calcium levels.

Cardiac output drops with burn shock.

Reasons: Due to loss of fluids and increased peripheral resistance (vasoconstriction from catecholamine release by the sympathetic nervous system).

Increased peripheral vascular resistance may occur after a burn injury.

Reason: This is a normal neurohormonal response to trauma.

Peripheral Circulation -- Shift from Central Venous Pool

A dramatic fall in BP occurs when a bedridden individual attempts to stand up.

> Reasons: From (1) shifting of the blood out of the central venous pool into the peripheral veins and (2) decreased stroke volume. This phenomenon is called orthostatic or postural hypotension.

Chapter 5: Pulmonary Circulation and Pulmonary Embolism

Pulmonary Circulation/ Blood Flow

Pulmonary blood flow is not uniformly distributed throughout the lungs.

> Reasons: Gravity dependence from regional differences in pulmonary vascular pressure and resistance.

Pulmonary circulation affects the blood composition supplying all organs.

> Reason: All CO goes through the lungs before entering the systemic circulation.

With mitral stenosis, pulmonary blood flow eventually decreases (which then decreases the systemic blood flow).

> Reason: Failure of the right ventricle.

Right ventricular failure develops with aortic stenosis.

Reason: Because of pulmonary congestion (resulting from increased pulmonary vascular pressures), pressures in the right chambers increase.

Symptoms of large-sized ventricular septal defects (VSD) may be delayed.

Reason: From the delayed decrease in pulmonary vascular pressures.

Symptoms of medium-sized VSDs occur earlier in premature infants than in full-term infants.

Reason: Pulmonary resistance decreases earlier in premature infants than in full-term infants.

Infants with medium-sized VSDs may have frequent respiratory infections.

Reason: This is secondary to the pulmonary congestion.

Pulmonary embolism (PE) results in increased pulmonary vascular resistance.

Reason: Reduction of the cross-sectional area of the pulmonary vascular bed.

Pulmonary embolism (PE) increases the right ventricular afterload.

Reason: Because of increased pulmonary vascular resistance.

Forced lung inflation causes increased right ventricular afterload.

Reason: The increased intrathoracic pressure compresses the pulmonary microcirculation.

Diffusion impairment occurs with pulmonary edema.

Reasons: From increased pulmonary capillary permeability or increased pulmonary vascular pressure.

Cardiac output increases as early as the fifth week of pregnancy.

Reasons: Function of reduced systemic vascular resistance and increased heart rate.

Pulmonary Embolism (PE) -- Anti-coagulation Treatment

Anticoagulation is a standard treatment for both deep venous thrombosis (DVT) and pulmonary embolism (PE).

Reason: Recurrence increases with delayed or inadequate anticoagulation.

Urokinase may be administered for pulmonary embolus.

> Reason: Urokinase directly converts plasminogen to plasmin.

Pulmonary Embolism (PE) -- Causes

Polycythemia can lead to PE.

> Reason: Increased viscosity of the blood predisposes to thrombi and/or emboli formation.

Venous stasis can lead to PE.

> Reason: Platelet and thrombin accumulate in the veins.

Factor V Leiden mutation, the most common cause of familial thromboembolism, can lead to PE.

> Reason: Factor V Leiden mutation causes a hypercoagulable state.

Raised venous pressure in HF can lead to PE.

> Reason: Increased viscosity of the blood.

Deficiencies (primary or acquired) in natural anticoagulants – protein C, protein S, and antithrombin III – are risk factors for PE.

Reason: Deficiencies of these natural anticoagulants can lead to venous thrombosis.

Compression of a vein by a tumor can lead to PE.

Reason: Increased viscosity of the blood.

The physical findings of hypotension, pulmonary edema, and cyanosis are red flags for individuals with leg pain and swelling.

Reasons: Hypotension, pulmonary edema, and cyanosis, in individuals with leg pain and swelling suggest possible diagnoses of PE, HF or dysrhythmias.

Pulmonary Embolism (PE) -- Complications

Hemodynamic compromise may occur with PE.

Reason: This may be due to large thrombi lodging at the bifurcation of the main pulmonary artery or the lobar branches.

Pulmonary embolism (PE) results in increased pulmonary vascular resistance.

Reason: Because of the reduction in the cross-sectional area of the pulmonary vascular bed.

Pulmonary embolism (PE) increases the right ventricular afterload.

Reason: From increased pulmonary vascular resistance.

In severe cases, PE can lead to right ventricular failure.

Reason: Due to a severe increase in afterload.

Pulmonary Embolism (PE) -- Diagnosis of

Pulmonary embolism (PE) is commonly the cause of death in hospitalized elderly patients.

Reason: Most hospitalized elderly patients are bedridden. Prolonged bed rest predisposes these patients to PE. In addition, diagnosis of PE is commonly missed.

Pulmonary embolism (PE) is a difficult diagnosis to make.

Reason: Poor sensitivity and specificity of the history taking and physical examination done on patients since most patients present with nonspecific signs and symptoms.

Pulmonary Embolism (PE) -- Chest radiograph

A chest radiograph is useful when diagnosing PE.

Reason: Most patients with PE have abnormal chest radiographs.

Pulmonary Embolism (PE) -- Consequences

Bronchoconstriction occurs with PE.

Reasons: The bronchoconstriction results in alveolar hypocarbia, hypoxia, and mediator release.

Pulmonary embolism (PE) can precipitate a syncopal attack.

Reason: PE interferes with CO.

Pulmonary Embolism (PE) -- Microemboli

Ventilation/ perfusion mismatch occur with septic shock.

Reasons: Pulmonary vasoconstriction and formation of pulmonary microemboli.

Pulmonary Embolism (PE) -- Physiology

Alveolar dead space increases with pulmonary embolus.

Reason: The affected part of the lung receives ventilation without perfusion.

Compensatory shunting occurs with pulmonary embolus.

Reason: The unaffected lung areas have to accommodate the entire CO.

Increased pulmonary extravascular water causes pulmonary edema.

Reasons: Because of increased pulmonary capillary permeability or increased pulmonary vascular pressure.

Pleuritic pain occurs with PE.

Reason: From an inflammatory reaction of the lung parenchyma.

Pulmonary Embolism (PE) -- Prevention of

If traveling for long periods of time, exercise at least every two hours.

Reason: To reduce risk of PE.

Drug holidays are no longer recommended for the treatment of Parkinson's disease with Levodopa.

> Reasons: Because of the risks of aspiration pneumonia, venous thrombosis, PE, and depression.

Pulmonary Embolism (PE) -- Risk Factors

Polycythemia vera increases the risk for PE.

> Reason: Due to hyperviscous blood.

Thrombosis formation above the knee has a poorer prognosis than thrombosis formation below the knee.

> Reasons: Thrombosis formation above the knee is associated with PE, MI and CVA.

Pulmonary Embolism (PE) -- Signs and Symptoms

Although PE is common and potentially lethal, the diagnosis is often missed.

> Reason: Patients with PE often present with nonspecific signs and symptoms.

Dyspnea may not always be present with PE.

Reason: Dyspnea may not be present while the patient is at rest.

Exercise can exaggerate the pleuritic pain from PE.

Reason: Because of the increased frequency of respirations with exercise.

Hypotension can occur with acute massive PE.

Reason: Hypotension is indicative of severe hemodynamic compromise.

Retrosternal pressure/ pain may occur with PE.

Reason: Due to associated myocardial ischemia.

Recurrent chest pain may occur after an MI.

Reasons: Recurrent chest pain, after an MI, may be caused by recurrent ischemia, reinfarction, pericarditis, subacute cardiac rupture, or PE.

Syncope can occur with acute massive PE.

Reason: Syncope is indicative of severe hemodynamic compromise.

Tachycardia may not always be present as a sign of PE.

Reason: Tachycardia may be either transient or relative.

Tachycardia can occur with PE.

Reason: To compensate for decreased oxygen supply.

Tachypnea may not always present as a symptom in PE.

Reason: Tachypnea may not be present at rest.

Wheezing may be heard in some patients with possible PE.

Reason: From reflex bronchoconstriction in the embolized area.

Syncope is a red flag for individuals with leg pain and swelling.

Reason: Syncope, with leg pain and swelling, suggest a possible diagnosis of PE or dysrhythmia.

Fever is a red flag for individuals with leg pain and swelling.

Reason: Fever, with leg pain and swelling, suggest a possible diagnosis of PE or systemic infection.

Chest pain is a red flag for individuals with leg pain and swelling.

Reason: Chest pain, with leg pain and swelling, suggest a possible diagnosis of PE or HF or dysrhythmia.

Dyspnea and tachypnea are red flags for individuals with leg pain and swelling.

> Reason: Dyspnea and tachypnea, with leg pain and swelling, suggest a possible diagnosis of PE or HF or dysrhythmia.

Pulmonary Embolism (PE) -- Treatment

Oxygen therapy is administered in the treatment of acute PE.

> Reason: Management of arterial hypoxemia, which is common among patients with acute PE.

Oxygen therapy is administered by nasal cannula or face mask in patients with acute PE.

> Reason: Oxygen therapy administration by nasal cannula or face mask is usually sufficient for keeping arterial oxyhemoglobin saturation at normal levels.

Mechanical administration of oxygen is usually not advisable in treating patients with acute PE.

> Reason: Mechanical delivery of oxygen can be detrimental to CO in right ventricular failure.

Streptokinase may be administered for pulmonary embolus.

Reason: Streptokinase binds to plasminogen and the complex breaks down fibrin clot.

When treating PE and infarction, a filter may be implanted in the inferior vena cava.

Reason: To prevent large thrombi from entering the lungs.

Chapter 6: Thromboembolism, Thrombophlebitis and Thrombosis

Thromboembolism or Chronic Thromboembolic Pulmonary HTN (CTEPH)

Oral anticoagulants are administered to patients with atrial fibrillation.

> Reason: To prevent thromboembolism or chronic thromboembolic pulmonary HTN (CTEPH).

Oral anticoagulants are administered to patients with cardiomyopathy.

> Reason: Also to prevent CTEPH.

Heparin may be administered to treat venous CTEPH in pregnant women.

> Reason: Pregnancy induces a hypercoagulable state that lasts about 10 to 11 months.

Surgery can increase the risk for venous CTEPH.

Reasons: Due to the activation of clotting factors and immobility/ prolonged bed rest.

Accidental trauma can increase the risk for venous CTEPH.

Reason: Because of the activation of clotting factors.

Thromboembolic disorders are a complication of atrial fibrillation.

Reason: As a result of venostasis (the blood pools in the atria which leads to the formation of small clots).

One should not rely on physical assessment alone to determine the presence of thromboembolism.

Reasons: It is the least reliable method; preferred methods include ultrasonography, venography and impedance plethysmography.

Thrombophlebitis -- Acute Superficial Venous Thrombosis (ASVT)

Thrombophlebitis is also called acute superficial venous thrombosis (ASVT).

Reasons: Due to the presence of both thrombotic and inflammatory components.

Thrombophlebitis (ASVT) is a common complication of pancreatic carcinoma.

Reason: Because of increased levels of thromboplastic factors in the blood.

Deep vein/venous thrombosis (DVT) can arise from ASVT.

Reason: As a consequence of ASVT extension into a deep vein at either the common femoral junction, the popliteal vein, or perforating veins.

Many healthcare practitioners do not actively manage ASVT.

Reason: Historically, ASVT was viewed as a benign disease.

Thrombosis -- Causes

Myeloproliferative disorders may predispose patients to both bleeding and thrombosis.

Reason: As a result of abnormal platelet function.

Thrombosis, ischemia, and infarction occur with sickle cell disease.

Reason: Masses of sickled red blood cells occlude blood vessels.

Thrombotic events occur with systemic lupus erythematosus.

Reason: The thrombotic events are secondary to lupus anticoagulants.

Atherosclerosis and thrombosis are causes of ischemic heart disease.

Reason: Decreased blood supply results in decreased oxygen.

Orally administered estrogen can increase thrombosis risk.

Reason: Estrogen's first pass metabolism in the liver leads to the production of increased levels of clotting factors.

Transdermal patches to administer 17-beta estradiol are recommended for persons with thromboembolic disease.

Reason: With transdermal patches, there is no first pass metabolism through the liver which increases the production of clotting factors.

Thrombosis occurs with polycythemia vera.

Reasons: Because of (1) increased blood viscosity, (2) thrombocytosis, and (3) platelet defects.

Nicotine increases the risk of thrombus formation in small blood vessels.

Reasons: Due to increased platelet adhesion and vasoconstriction.

Increased incidence of thromboembolic phenomena can result from pain.

Reasons: Because pain triggers (1) increased platelet adhesiveness, (2) diminished fibrinolysis and (3) activation of the coagulation cascade.

Pregnant women are at increased risk of thrombotic complications.

Reasons: Due to increased platelet adhesiveness and decreased fibrinolysis during pregnancy.

Thrombosis -- Complications

Thromboemboli are a cause of ischemic heart disease.

Reason: Decreased blood supply results in decreased oxygen supply.

Thrombosis -- Coronary

Death can occur from Kawasaki Disease during the convalescent phase (10-40 days after the onset of fever).

> Reason: Most often from acute MI due to acute coronary artery thrombosis.

Thrombosis -- Deep Vein/Venous Thrombosis (DVT)

Venous incompetence with reflux and backflow of blood occur as a long-term complication of DVT.

> Reason: The venous incompetence is the result of damage to venous valves.

Hydrostatic pressure increases below the area damaged by DVT.

> Reason: Damage to venous valves causes venous incompetence.

Thrombi in deep veins (such as the ones in the calf or thigh muscles) are more dangerous than thrombi in superficial veins.

> Reason: The deep veins are not only larger but they also communicate more directly to the heart and lungs.

Thrombi in veins close to the ankle are not as dangerous as those above the knee.

> Reason: Thrombi in veins close to the ankle rarely embolize.

The tendency of free-flowing blood to clot increases after fractures and surgical operations which result in immobilization of the lower limbs.

> Reason: If a limb is suddenly immobilized, and remains so for more than 48 hours, the blood flow through that limb flows very slowly and results in stasis.

Compression stockings should be worn on airplane flights longer than two hours.

> Reason: Due to severe restrictions in walking during long flights, asymptomatic DVT has been noted in as much of 10% of travelers.

The development of thrombosis is common in diabetes mellitus.

> Reasons: From an enhanced coagulation process and impaired fibrinolysis.

Antiphospholipid antibody syndrome is an inherited disease that predisposes individuals to DVT.

Reason: Due to hypercoagulability of the blood.

Antithrombin 3 deficiency is an inherited disease that predisposes individuals to DVT.

Reason: Also due to hypercoagulability of the blood.

Factor V Leiden is an inherited disease that predisposes individuals to DVT.

Reason: Because of the hypercoagulability of the blood.

Protein C deficiency is an inherited disease that predisposes individuals to DVT.

Reason: Also because of the hypercoagulability of the blood.

Protein S deficiency is an inherited disease that predisposes individuals to DVT.

Reason: Hypercoagulability of the blood.

With DVT, the calf muscle can become edematous.

Reason: Chronic congestion of the calf muscle results from obstruction of the vein.

A negative D-dimer test is an important diagnostic finding.

Reason: It rules out DVT in individuals who are unlikely to have DVT.

Compression ultrasonography may be utilized in the evaluation of symptomatic individuals with suspected DVT.

Reason: The compression ultrasonography permits detection of above-the-knee thrombosis.

A patient in traction is encouraged to perform ankle and foot exercises (within the limits of traction therapy).

Reason: To prevent DVT resulting from venous stasis.

Streptokinase may be administered for DVT.

Reasons: Streptokinase binds to plasminogen and the complex breaks down fibrin clots.

Anticoagulant therapy is administered to patients diagnosed with DVT.

Reasons: To (1) prevent PE, (2) reestablish venous patency, (3) restore valvular function of veins, and (4) prevent postphlebitic syndrome.

Thrombosis -- Origin

Thrombosis formation above the knee has a poorer prognosis than thrombosis formation below the knee.

Reason: Thrombosis formation above the knee is associated with PE.

Thrombosis -- Prevention

Anticoagulation therapy may be administered to treat pulmonary HTN.

Reason: To reduce the likelihood of venous thrombus formation.

Thrombosis -- Splenic Vein

Among patients with variceal hemorrhage, higher rates of bleeding are reported in those with left-sided portal HTN.

Reason: Because of splenic vein thrombosis.

Thrombosis -- Thrombolytics

Thrombolytics may cause bleeding.

Reason: Thrombolytics increase fibrinolytic activity.

Thrombosis -- Treatment

Treatment of a thrombus must be prompt.

Reasons: To (1) reduce the risk of thrombus extension, (2) minimize thrombus propagation and (3) reduce the risk of post-thrombotic syndrome.

Warfarin is contraindicated during pregnancy.

Reason: Warfarin is teratogenic if taken by pregnant women at 6 to12 weeks of gestation.

Heparin is the initial treatment of choice in the management of a thrombus.

Reasons: Heparin has (1) rapid onset and (2) reduces the risk of further thromboembolic events.

Niacin can reverse some endothelial cell dysfunction that contributes to thrombosis associated with hypercholesterolemia and atherosclerosis.

Reasons: Niacin boosts the secretion of tissue plasminogen activator and lowers plasma fibrinogen.

Thrombosis -- Venous

A venous clot gradually occludes a vein.

> Reason: A venous clot arises from a low-flow portion of a vein behind a valve and subsequently propagates proximally. Note: Venous thrombi rarely form at the sites of vascular disruption.

Venous thrombi most often originate around valves or in muscular sinuses.

> Reason: Prevalence of stasis (slow blood flow) in those areas.

Venous thrombi form where diminished blood supply is available to the lining of the vein segments involved.

> Reason: Diminished blood supply results from stasis (slow blood flow).

Venous thrombi consist primarily of fibrin and trapped red blood cells, but relatively few platelets.

> Reason: Venous thrombi form under low shear.

Venous thrombi appear red.

> Reason: Due to high red blood cell content.

Chapter 7: Disseminated Intravascular Coagulation

Disseminated Intravascular Coagulation (DIC) -- Blood/ Serum

Hemolysis (intravascular or otherwise) can lead to disseminated intravascular coagulation (DIC).

Reason: Due to liberation of tissue factors.

Acute promyelocytic leukemia can lead to DIC.

Reason: Also because of the liberation of tissue factors.

Fat embolism can lead to DIC.

Reason: Also from the liberation of tissue factors.

Bleeding time is prolonged with DIC.

Reason: Split fibrin products from DIC inhibit platelet function.

Disseminated Intravascular Coagulation (DIC) -- Cardiovascular

Disseminated intravascular coagulation (DIC) involves simultaneous microvascular clotting and hemorrhage in organ systems.

Reasons: From (1) depletion of clotting factors and (2) excessive fibrinolysis.

Aortic aneurysm can lead to DIC.

Reason: Endothelial damage.

Hemolytic uremic syndrome can lead to DIC.

Reason: Also because of endothelial damage.

Acute glomerulonephritis can lead to DIC.

Reason: Also from endothelial damage.

Kasabach-Merritt syndrome can lead to DIC.

Reasons: Vascular malformations and decreased blood flow.

Disseminated Intravascular Coagulation (DIC) -- Critical Illness

All critically ill patients are at risk for developing DIC.

> Reasons: Many are in physiological disequilibrium; procoagulant effects exist with hypovolemia, hypotension, hypoxia, and acidosis.

Occasionally, fresh frozen plasma is required for patients with acute myelogenous leukemia (AML), particularly in AML patients with DIC.

> Reason: To correct coagulopathies.

Disseminated Intravascular Coagulation (DIC) -- Infections

Rocky Mountain spotted fever can lead to DIC.

> Reason: Due to endothelial damage.

Disseminated Intravascular Coagulation (DIC) -- Neoplasms

Neoplasms (particularly mucinous adenocarcinomas) can lead to DIC.

Reason: Because of the liberation of tissue factors.

Disseminated Intravascular Coagulation (DIC) -- Pregnancy Complications

Abruptio placentae can lead to DIC.

Reason: From the liberation of tissue factors.

Amniotic fluid embolism can lead to DIC.

Reason: Also due to the liberation of tissue factors.

A retained dead fetus can lead to DIC.

Reason: Also because of the liberation of tissue factors.

A second trimester abortion can lead to DIC.

Reason: Also from the liberation of tissue factors.

All patients with hydatidiform moles should be screened for DIC.

Reason: The molar tissue releases factors with fibrinolytic activity.

Disseminated Intravascular Coagulation (DIC) -- Physiology/ Pathophysiology

Obstruction of small-size and mid-size vessels by thrombi occurs with DIC.

> Reason: As a consequence of the widespread systemic activation of coagulation.

Cellular injury or lysis is involved in the development of DIC.

> Reason: Tissue phospholipid is released into the bloodstream, triggering intrinsic pathway activity.

All organ systems may fail or become dysfunctional with DIC.

> Reasons: Because of bleeding into tissue spaces and/or ischemia caused by thrombosis.

Disseminated Intravascular Coagulation (DIC) -- Trauma/ Acute Conditions

Burns can lead to DIC.

> Reason: From liberation of tissue factors.

Head injury can lead to DIC.

Reason: Also due to the liberation of tissue factors.

Frostbite can lead to DIC.

Reason: Also because of the liberation of tissue factors.

Gunshot wounds can lead to DIC.

Reason: Also from the liberation of tissue factors.

Disseminated Intravascular Coagulation (DIC) -- Treatment

Transfusion of cryoprecipitate is included in the treatment of DIC.

Reason: To treat hypofibrinogenemia.

Transfusion of blood products, such as packed red blood cells and platelets, are included in the treatment of DIC.

Reason: To correct clotting factor deficiencies.

Cryoprecipitate, not fresh frozen plasma, is administered to patients with DIC.

Reason: Cryoprecipitate contains concentrated factor VIII, vWF and fibrinogen; fresh frozen plasma contains all factors but only small amounts of fibrinogen.

Plasma or platelet substitution therapy is not always necessary based only on laboratory results indicating low levels of platelets and coagulation factors.

Reason: They are indicated if there is active bleeding or there is a risk for bleeding (e.g., after an invasive procedure).

Appendix: Abbreviations

ACE Inhibitor – Angiotensin-Converting Enzyme Inhibitor
ADH – Antidiuretic Hormone
ANA – Antinuclear Antibody
ARB – Angiotensin Receptor Blocker
ARDS – Adult or Acute Respiratory Distress Syndrome
ASVT – Acute Superficial Venous Thrombosis
BP – Blood Pressure
CBC – Complete Blood Count
CPP – Cerebral Perfusion Pressure
CO – Cardiac Output
COPD – Chronic Obstructive Pulmonary Disease
CTEPH – Chronic Thromboembolic Pulmonary Hypertension
CT Scan – Computerized Tomography Scan
CVA – Cerebrovascular Accident
DIC – Disseminated Intravascular Coagulation
DKA – Diabetic Ketoacidosis
DVT – Deep Vein/Venous Thrombosis
EKG – Electrocardiogram
GFR – Glomerular Filtration Rate
HF – Heart Failure
HIV – Human Immunodeficiency Virus

ICP – Intracranial Pressure
IPAH – Idiopathic Pulmonary Arterial Hypertension
HTN – Hypertension
MAO Inhibitor – Monoamine Oxidase Inhibitor
MI – Myocardial Infarction
OA – Osteoarthritis
PAD – Peripheral Arterial Disease
PAH –Pulmonary Arterial Hypertension
PCWP – Pulmonary Capillary Wedge Pressure
PE – Pulmonary Embolism
PFO –Patent Foramen Ovale
PFT – Pulmonary Function Testing
PIH – Pregnancy-Induced Hypertension
PH – Pulmonary Hypertension
PPH – Primary Pulmonary Hypertension
POTS – Postural Orthostatic Tachycardia Syndrome
PVD – Peripheral Vascular Disease
RF – Renal Failure
SIRS – Systemic Inflammatory Response Syndrome
SOB – Shortness Of Breath
V/Q Scan – Ventilation-Perfusion Scan
VSD –Ventricular Septal Defect

About The Authors

[illegible]

[illegible]

About The Authors

James L. Jordan, PhD, PhD, and Deovina N. Jordan, PhD, MD, celebrate more than 80 years of combined remarkable experiences in their professional lives. They are noted for their significant achievements and outstanding successes in healthcare, science, management, and higher education (with senior professorial ranks). Dr. James L. Jordan and Dr. Deovina N. Jordan have authored several books and many peer reviewed journal articles. They are developing scientific theories. Dr. James L. Jordan and Dr. Deovina N. Jordan have been highlighted in over 20 editions of Marquis Who's Who (in America, West, World, Medicine, Healthcare, Education, and Worldwide Lifetime Achievement).

Dr. James L. Jordan and Dr. Deovina N. Jordan live in a farm in the mountains with their two Yorkshire terriers and abundant wildlife. They share a love for wisdom literature and nature.

About The Book

This book addresses both "whats" and "whys", and "whats" and "hows" and has been arranged not only by topic but also according to statements. The "what" statements are mentioned first. Then the "why" or "how" statements follow. The authors acknowledge a certain lack of continuity that would be present if only facts or "whats" are presented. To the authors' knowledge, this is the first time such an attempt to systematically address "whats" and their "whys" or "hows" have been made. Considering the time utilized and the efforts expended to obtain the information included in this book, along with the vast sea of information which needed to be reviewed in order to glean these pearls of understanding, this is quite understandable. Few people would have gone on a thirty year journey, surveying thousands of documents, without knowing where it would lead them.

The published literature on healthcare abounds in presentations of information focused on a plethora of facts. The authors wholeheartedly believe that these sources of information are invaluable in healthcare practice and understanding. Also, other publications often address current healthcare theories and hypotheses. These will help healthcare practitioners understand what the current thought and research trends are. However, healthcare theories and hypotheses are not addressed in this book as they often change with the times.

This book is about the "Whats," "Whys" and "Hows" or Rationales of Cardiology. Book One focuses on the Cardiovascular System and is specifically about Blood Flow; Blood Pressure, Hypertension (HTN) (Different Types) and Hypotension; Blood Supply, Blood Volume and Circulation; Peripheral Circulation, Deep Vein/Venous Thrombosis, Peripheral Arterial Disease, and Peripheral Vascular Disease; Pulmonary Circulation and Pulmonary Embolism; Thromboembolism, Thrombophlebitis and Thrombosis; and Disseminated Intravascular Coagulation. Pulmonary circulation was included as part of the cardiovascular system. Some topics may be repeated in different sections due to the overlap of disorders when discussing the cardiovascular system. Topics within the chapters are arranged alphabetically. The information presented in this book reflects the latest in literature as of publication date.

Finally, this is not a book written to provide medical, nursing, or any other healthcare advice. This book is in no way a substitute for well-trained healthcare professionals practicing in their fields of expertise.

Other Books Written By The Authors

God: Answering the Mysteries of God, God's Existence, the Trinity, and God's Love; and How to Have a Personal Relationship with God

Link to Ebook: **https://www.amazon.com/dp/B082RNRVBF**

The Universe is Not Dying: A unified physics theory explaining the mysteries of dimensions, space, strings, matter, energy, light, time, particle spin, wave formation, black holes, quasars, and the energy-matter cycle

Link to Ebook: **https://www.amazon.com/dp/B083DP6MVC**

Drs. Jordan's Fables: Book One

Link to Ebook: **https://www.amazon.com/dp/B084FZH9DY**

Drs. Jordan's Fables: Book Two

Ebook link: **https://www.amazon.com/dp/B084WNG8W8**

Thus Says The Lord God

Ebook link: **https://www.amazon.com/dp/B085BLSH23**

Drs. Jordan's Fables: Book Three

Ebook link: **https://www.amazon.com/dp/B085QBWXHP**

Thus Say The Biblical Prophets And Apostles: Volume I

Ebook link: **https://www.amazon.com/dp/B08689G32J**

Thus Say The Biblical Prophets And Apostles: Volume II

Ebook link: **https://www.amazon.com/dp/B086JFY6KB**

What Is A Good Husband?

Ebook link: **https://www.amazon.com/dp/B0871T5ZQQ**

The Lost Books Of Wisdom

Ebook link: **https://www.amazon.com/dp/B087BF3WV6**

The Ancient Wisdom Of The West

Ebook link: **https://www.amazon.com/dp/B087Q566F7**

Christian Faith In The Age Of Disbelief And Unbelief: Attaining, Growing And Maintaining The Christian Faith Needed For Salvation

Ebook link: **https://www.amazon.com/dp/B0881J6LM3**

Drs. Jordan's Proverbial Wit And Wisdom From The Animal Kingdom

Ebook link: **https://www.amazon.com/dp/B088F6RSQ7**

Many peer reviewed journal articles

Made in the USA
Monee, IL
05 November 2026

67811169R00105